Birth of a Teenager
an owner's manual

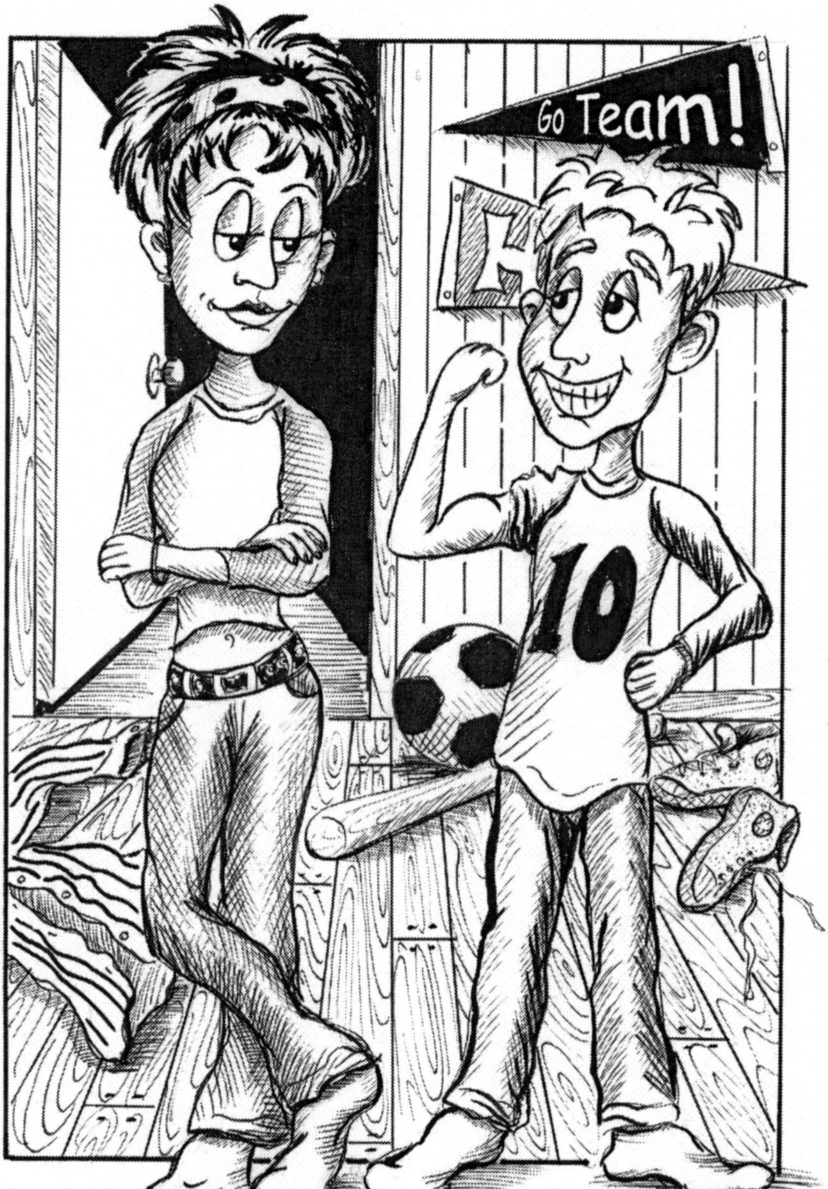

written by Corie Goodson MPH CHES

illustrated by Julie M. Malfitano

First published by Dog Ear Publishing
4010 W. 86th Street, Ste H
Indianapolis, IN 46268
www.dogearpublishing.net

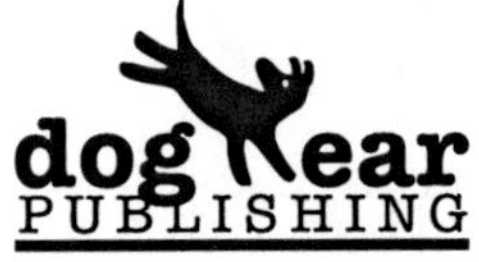

ISBN: 1-59858-086-8

This book is printed on acid-free paper.

Printed in the United States of America

Corie Goodson's Birth of a Teenager is a great resource for teenagers and their parents and provides a realistic approach to good nutrition. In addition to offering a wealth of information about the importance of incorporating healthy foods into our diets, Goodson includes easy to follow recipes to get readers started on the road to a healthier lifestyle. Goodson's approach is refreshing through her use of humor and understandable language, making the book both educational and entertaining. Goodson's passion is contagious, leaving readers with a renewed energy about a new outlook on the importance and value of making good nutritional choices. Goodson helps combat the unhealthy habits cultivated by our fast food culture and Birth of a Teenager is a must read!

- *Embracing Change* Magazine

This refreshing book is packed from cover to cover with realistic solutions and advice for our youth's health-related concerns. In an upcoming generation of body conscious yet often unhealthy tweens and teens, Birth of a Teenager brilliantly addresses the uniqueness of each individual as well as how to achieve optimal health. As the parent of a tween and a health care professional, I consider this a must read!

Kathy Moore, RN, BS, CHES

Birth of a Teenager is an upbeat informative book that is invaluable in understanding how we can help our teenagers control some of the ups and downs of the teen years. It contains reliable facts and sensible lifestyle changes which are applicable for teens as well as adults. The focus on healthy lifestyles, not calorie and carb numbers, is a refreshing message. I learned small changes that can have a large impact to improve my family's health and wellness. It is nice to read a "health" book which also gives you recipes. This is a must read for every teenager and his/her family. Where was this book when I was a teenager?

Tamara Moulton, mother of a teen and tween

I loved how Birth of a Teenager addressed questions my friends and I have but don't know who to ask. The recipes are great and satisfy my sweet cravings and most are fast and easy with little clean-up. Sometimes making and eating healthy food is hard as so much work goes into it. These recipes use common ingredients we have at home. I like how the book addresses how food will affect your life. I like the way the author explains why things are bad and why we should eat certain things. If you eat healthier your mood improves and you won't be irritable. Now when my body is run down, I know why. "Junk in equals junk out" reminds me to eat healthy to improve my energy and health while reducing my mood swings during a time when my body is changing and growing so fast.

Christina Moulton, age 15

Three cheers for "Birth of a Teenager"! I have been in the business of health education for 11 years; I constantly hear "if I only knew then what I know now" or "I wish I'd taken better care of myself". I've also heard many adults admit they do not know how to cook and don't even feel comfortable enough in a kitchen to experiment with cooking. This book can solve both problems. Give this book to all the young people you know…learn together, cook together and get healthy together!

Tracy Hadfield Hubbard, RD
www.healthylifesolutions.org

Table of Contents

Life…is drawing without an eraser but experience can be a great teacher if you let it.

—Unknown

Dedication

To my family and friends who continue to support and inspire me.

To Julie Malfitano, without her vision and wonderful talent, this book wouldn't be the same.

And to my 2 dogs Mika and Kona who don't let me forget that there is fun to be had every day!

A note to the Girls

Being a teenager can be tough. It's a time when your body is changing, your mind is starting to think differently and you are sort of in limbo between being a kid and an adult. No one said it was going to be easy, but the good news is, you can minimize the collateral damage it takes to grow up. All it takes is a little common sense, a good sense of humor and a whole lot of patience. This age is also an exciting time of discovery and possibility. The world is at your feet and you can do and become anything you want to. Growing up will happen in its own time. Focusing on the positive things will help put you on the path to whatever success you desire.

Now I know about as well as anyone that many girls tend to compare themselves to other girls and worry about body image. No one wants to be different or stand out too much. However, it's important to note that looking one way or another does not always equate to being healthy. Especially if you obsess about the things you cannot change.

For example, there is a difference between being "thin" and "fit" and often times being fit means you may not be as thin as some other girls you know. Not to worry, health is definitely a better place to be. Anyway, here's a little secret…those models you see in the glam mag's don't look like that in real life! Body image is important, but putting too much emphasis on trying to achieve a look that doesn't fit your body type and profile will only be frustrating and cause undue stress.

The wonderful thing about being human is that we are all different and unique. What is most important to remember is who you are inside. Your friends like you for who you are, not what you look like on the outside. Be kind to yourself, respect your body and yourself by taking care of YOU and you will be just fine. How boring would life be if everyone wore the same size, had the same hair and eye color and liked the same things anyway?

In this book we'll talk a little about exercise and its benefits as well as why and how you should be eating healthy. And, if you want to lose a few pounds, we'll talk about how you can accomplish that without compromising your health, metabolism or your good nature. You can use this book as an informational read or a cookbook. I hope you'll do both.

Read on girls and remember to have fun.

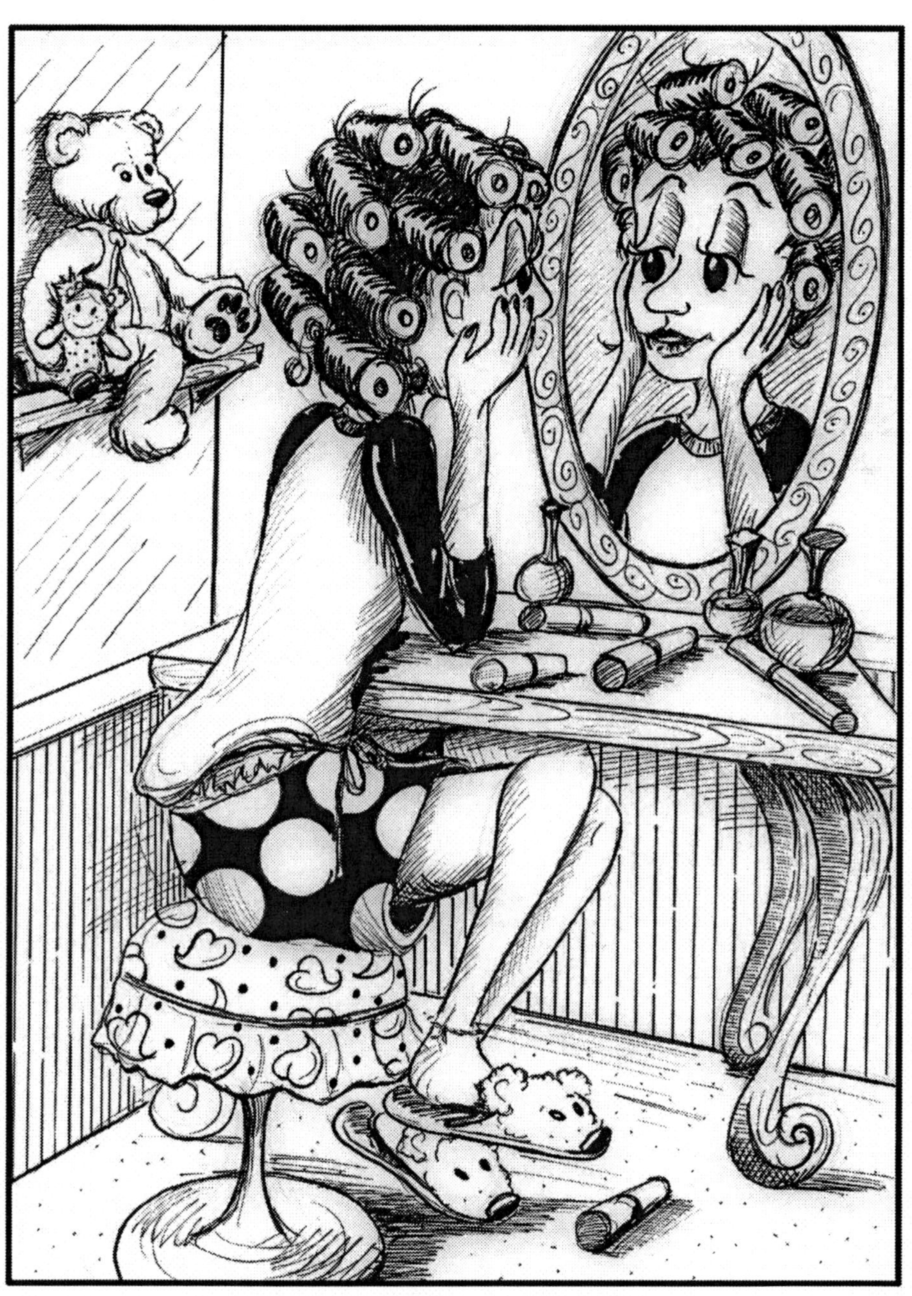

"Mirror, mirror on the wall . . ."

A note to the Boys

Growing up takes a lot of energy. Consequently you probably eat a lot more food than the rest of your family. Simply due to your genetic make up you have an advantage over the girls in that you can eat and eat and probably not gain any weight, at least not during your growing teen years. By nature, you go through a huge growth spurt between the tween and teen years. This growth spurt requires a lot of calories to build body mass, fill out and up.

It's important that you fuel that growth but it's also an important time for you to have the best nutrition you can. It's not okay to eat anything you want if it means nutritional deficiency in favor of lots of calories. In case you haven't noticed, the average portion size can now feed a family of four. What used to be a 1/4lb. burger has now tripled in size along with the super sized doses of artery clogging French fries, onion rings, sodas, and shakes.

These unreasonable portion sizes we have gotten used to have literally created a national epidemic of undernourished yet overfed people. As teenage boys you may not feel or see the effects of it yet, but the rising statistics of obesity, heart disease, high blood pressure and hypercholesterolemia (a fancy way of saying high cholesterol) are telling a different story.

You can help change the statistics by making some adjustments in what you eat and how you go about your day. Believe it or not, close to 80% of the state of your health now and in the future can be determined by what you eat and how you live.

I hope you give your creative side the chance to experiment in the kitchen and try some of these recipes also. Besides, truth be told, girls love it when a guy can cook!

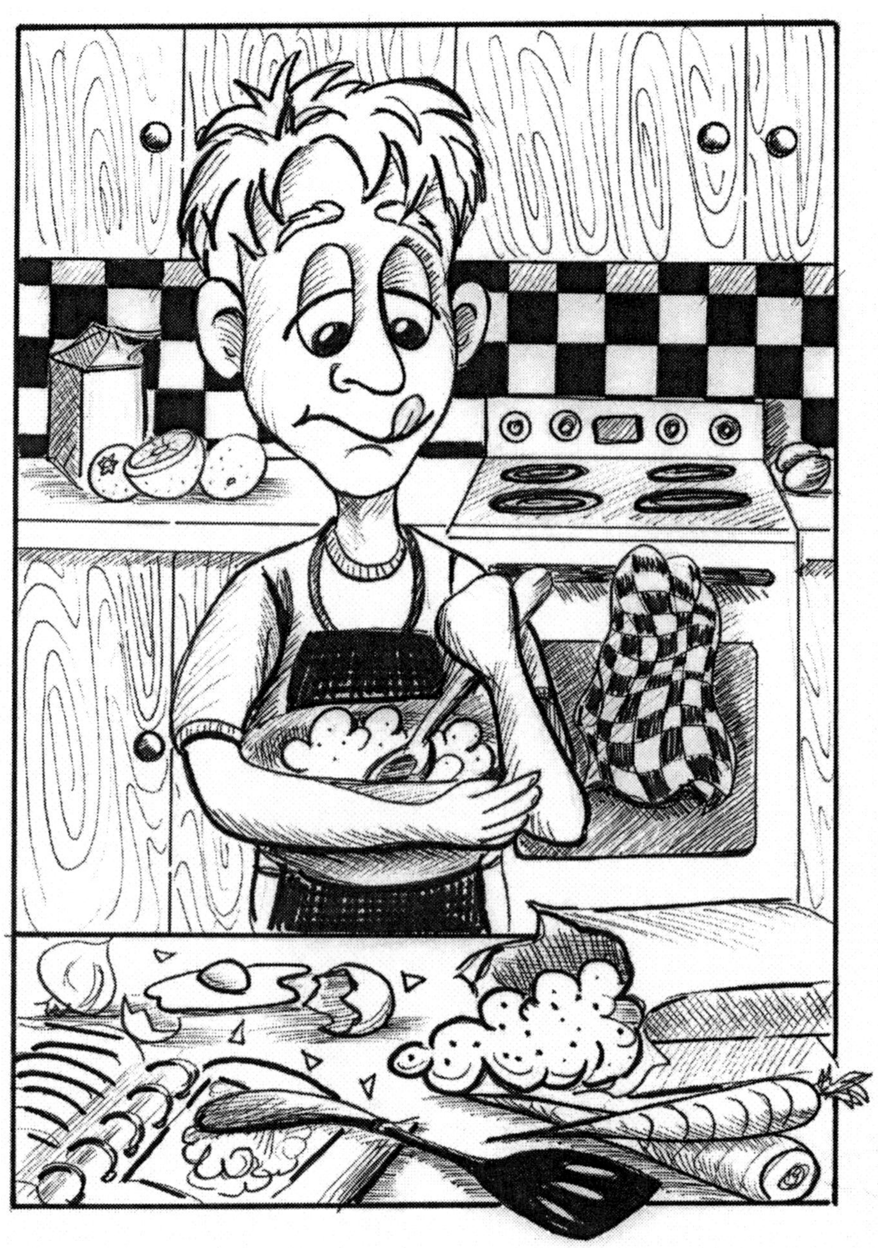

A note to the Parents

Being the quintessential health advocate that I am, I could not let this edition go unwritten. The current statistics on the state of the nation's health are truly alarming. With 1 in 3 Americans doomed to cancer in their lifetime (Am. Cancer Society) and 1.5 million Americans having heart attacks every year, it is only the tip of the iceberg. This is clearly a trend that has to be reversed if future generations are going to thrive not just survive.

The fundamental problem stems from all the "fake" and over-processed foods manufactured today for our convenience. Combine that with the huge portion sizes we have become accustomed to and the lack of physical activity that has been replaced by spectator sports, satellite dishes and reality TV, and we have a problem. Let's stop a moment to ponder this new phenomenon called reality TV. Does anyone really think this is reality? We were not meant to watch our lives but to live them, experience them in real time and enjoy all that this grand earth has to offer. We need to put down the remote, stop watching life go by and start actively living it.

All the ingredients for healthful living have already been given yet science keeps trying to improve upon what is already perfect. The sooner we realize that we can't fool Mother Nature the better off we and our children will be. We now have all the low-fat, no fat, artificial, low and no carb products on the market we can handle, yet obesity has doubled over the last 20 years and heart disease, stroke, cancer and degenerative disease statistics continue to rise. Unfortunately, all the genetic engineering and pharmaceutical advancements cannot compare to or improve upon the tools that nature has already provided for us to maintain good health. It's time to take back control and get back to the basics. Our health and the health of future generations depend on it.

We have to come a long way now to reverse the damage that has already been done, but I believe that small changes can add up to big results over time. With some simple modifications in what we eat, how we prepare food and how we go about or daily lives we can reverse these grim statistics and truly become a healthier nation. In some cases we need to stop obsessing about what we do eat and focus on what we are not eating enough of.

I hope you will use this book as an informational read as well as get in the kitchen with your kids. The recipes are healthful but not fanatical and they are easy to make. You can find all the ingredients at your neighborhood grocery store with the possible exception of organic meats and dairy products. I hope you take the time to purchase these options after reading the reasons why they are so important for you and your family. After all, family time is one of the healthiest ideas I can think of.

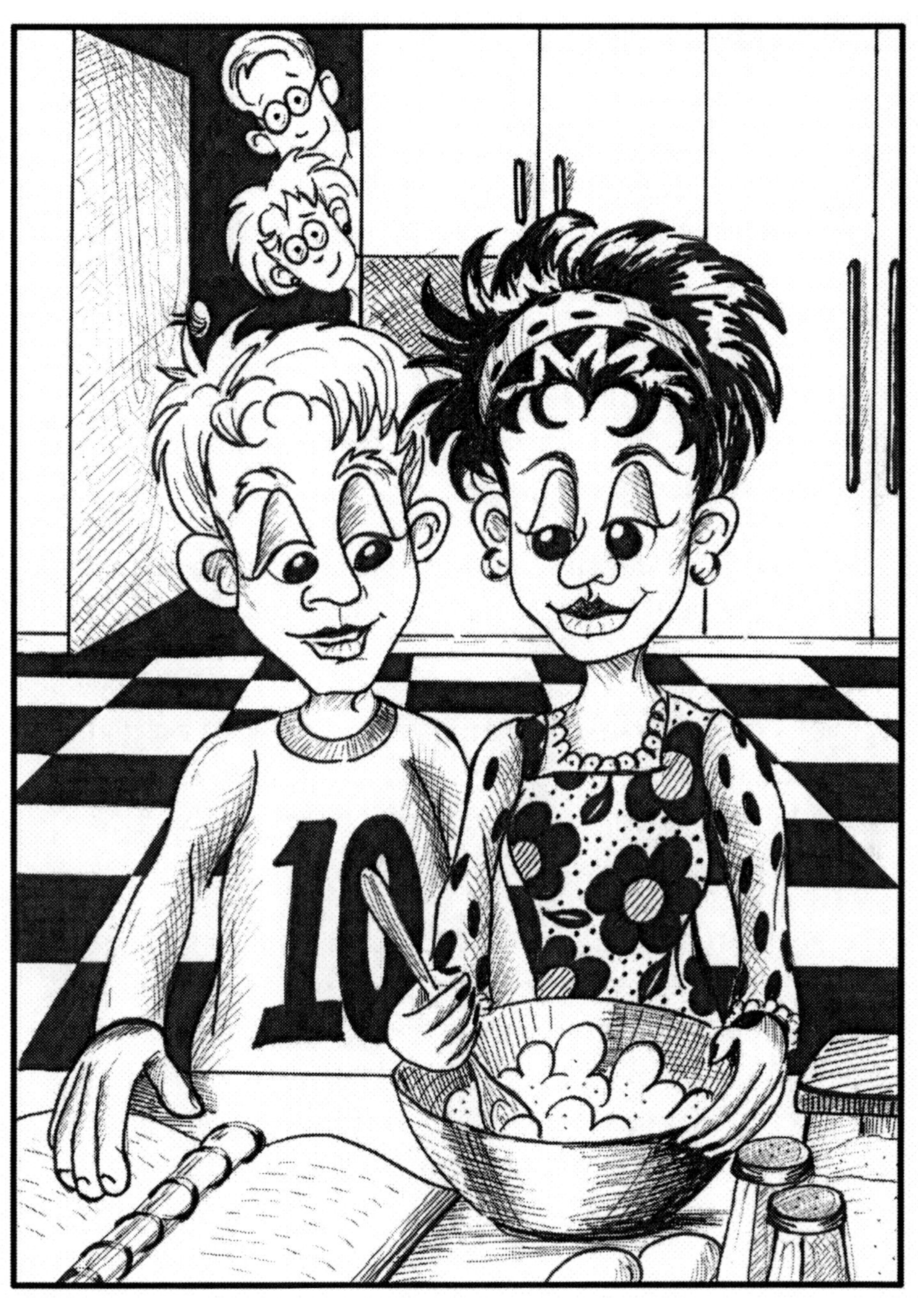

Disclaimer

Since not everyone uses cow's milk, note that any recipe calling for milk as an ingredient can be substituted with any milk product you use such as soy, almond or rice without really any change in taste or outcome.

Since oven temperatures vary, recommended cooking times may vary also. It is advised that products be checked frequently for doneness.

Altitude may affect time and temperature also, so baking times in particular are recommendations only.

Some of the recipes have been modified to be healthier versions of the originals. Emphasis was placed on using wholesome natural ingredients which in moderation are a much better alternative to the prepackaged processed choices on the market today.

The health information provided in this book is designed to help you understand certain concepts and trends and is not intended to diagnose or treat any conditions. If a medical condition exists, seek medical attention. Do not rely on self-diagnosis or attempt to treat yourself with supplements or over the counter preparations.

Introduction

It has been said that we do not have a vitamin deficiency, we have a whole food deficiency. There is power in whole food that can help your body stay strong and healthy without having to rely on fragmented vitamin supplementation.

Although I believe that eating a diet rich in a variety of fruits, vegetables and whole grains is our best bet for optimal health, the reality is that we can't or won't do it everyday. Another challenge we as consumers face is the lack of nutritional quality of some of the food choices on the market today. Unfortunately, some of the produce we buy has been harvested from nutritionally depleted or over-used soil which in turn causes the produce to be less nutritious than we would like. Also, much of it has to be picked before it is completely ripe in order to ensure its integrity during transport.

The main problem with this is that most of the nutrient content of fruits and veggies becomes available the last few days of the ripening cycle. So, if it is picked before it is ripe, it has not reached its full nutrient potential. Over half of the nutrition can be lost after about 7 days off the vine, branch or tree. In addition, the live enzymes found in raw fruits and veggies that are so beneficial to our health are destroyed by cooking.

So you can see the dilemma. In light of all of the barriers we face trying to get the best foods for ourselves and our families, most of us could use a little more dietary insurance. Recognizing this, we have traditionally turned to vitamins since this is what we have learned to do for generations. Unfortunately, they often leave us with false dietary support.

The one product I can wholeheartedly recommend to bridge the gap between what we know we need but just can't get for one reason or another is Juice Plus+®. Juice Plus+® is the essence of 17 vine ripened, raw fruits, vegetables and grains that have been juiced and then by a proprietary process put into capsule, gummie, or chewable form. It is the most researched whole food based nutritional product in the world and because it is not a "vitamin supplement" which is derived from individual nutrients that have been isolated, you receive the benefit of its full nutritional support. Our bodies recognize fruits and veggies in their whole form much better than individual vitamins that have been extracted from a food source or artificially manufactured. This is because fruits and veggies in their natural state offer thousands of vitamins, minerals and phytonutrients that work synergistically together to provide the nutritional benefits of all of the nutrients contained in each of the individual fruits and veggies. There is no disputing the fact that individual vitamin supplementation may be necessary for therapeutic reasons due to a diagnosed deficiency during short durations of time, but they really should not be used as a self prescribed regimen every day.

Lastly, to maintain a healthy diet and understand the values you find on labels, there are a few guidelines to note:

Your cholesterol intake should stay at or below 300 mg per day.

Your fat intake should not exceed 20–25% of your total calories per day.

Your salt intake should not exceed 1 tsp. per day or (2400 mg.)

I did not list calorie, carb, protein, or fat values for each recipe on purpose. The guidelines above give you a bench mark to shoot for and the recipes you will see in this book generally follow those guidelines with the exception of some of the desserts. As we know, dessert should not be considered a dietary staple anyway. It's not about counting every calorie or carb. That concept is so overrated it has spurred an entire revolution. I want the focus of this book to be more about healthier living rather than individual numbers. I believe that if you follow a healthy eating plan and lifestyle it transcends the obsession society has on these individual numbers. It's simply about getting back to basics.

To your health!

Corie Goodson MPH, CHES

Where does the RDA fit in?

Simply talking about protein, carbohydrates, fat and the RDA can be a snooze. However, if you weren't interested in your health you probably wouldn't have bought this book. No one can really completely appreciate what it means to eat healthy if they don't have a basic understanding of the various nutrients in foods and the body's requirements for them.

To say the least, nutrition information seems to be an ever-evolving ever-changing science. Anyone who tells you they know everything there is to know about it is probably suspect. In any given week we are told something which then gets contradicted the following week. What we accept as truth today may be questioned or disproved tomorrow. There is fundamental knowledge about health that does not change, but new discoveries are made every day that question what we believe. Because of this, it's often difficult to know how to proceed and what is truly best for our health. Unless you truly are an expert in the field it's hard to get it all right. When in doubt, seeking the advice of a professional is always a good idea.

Based on what researchers have discovered, experts have made specific recommendations for several nutrients. The most recognized is the RDA or Recommended Daily Allowance. The RDA is intended to provide minimum requirements needed to prevent deficiencies. What is important to note about this is that the RDA is simply a recommendation. In any case, the RDA specifies recommendations for protein, 11 vitamins and 7 minerals. It does not include recommendations for carbohydrate, fat, or fiber although there are some guidelines for those proportions based on percentages of calories consumed and they differ by age groups. Obviously there are many more nutrients that are not even considered in the recommendations.

What I want to have you understand about this is that these are not requirements, nor are they minimum intakes, they are simply what they are, recommendations. What this means to you is that the numbers for any given nutrient have been set high enough so that almost everyone, even those who have higher than average requirements, get enough nutrients to promote good health. However, the National Academy of Sciences' Food and Nutrition Board, which is responsible for setting the RDAs, emphasizes that the RDA's are designed to measure the nutritional adequacy of a population's diet, not an individual's (Webb & Smith, Foods for Better Health, 1995).

That said, this book is not designed to provide you with each individual nutrient value in the recipes. Most people just want to know what foods they should be including in their diets and why. That is what this book is about. Forget the fancy designer premanufactured foods and counting every protein and fat gram. This book is about getting back to the basics and getting back in the kitchen so that we can take control of what goes into our recipes and in our mouths. I hope to show you that it doesn't have to be complicated or a half day project to eat healthier. That said, there are recipes in the book that may not be considered "healthful" but are made with natural, not artificial, ingredients that the body recognizes, which are ultimately better choices than their premanufactured counterparts. A little common sense really does go a long way. Obviously cookies, Alfredo sauce, and desserts are not health foods and should be eaten in moderation. The recipes also don't cater to any one way of eating. Everyone has different tastes and will enjoy some recipes and not like others. That's the beauty of being unique. This book is designed to create awareness and a bit of experimentation.

The goal is to start you on the path to better eating habits that can help you transition into an even healthier plant-based diet. Many experts believe that in order to really promote better health we need our diet to be at least 75% plant-based, with animal products only comprising 10% of total calories consumed. This book does not accomplish that, but it is a place to start. Don't be afraid to modify the recipes to suit your likes. Cooking is an art and should be explored. Be creative! I sincerely hope you have fun with this and learn a little something along the way that will propel you into a healthier future.

Now let's get cooking and have some fun!

The importance of breakfast

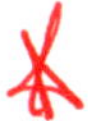Skipping breakfast could very well be one of the biggest nutritional mistakes anyone can make. I know, some people just can't imagine eating early in the day. That's okay, even having something light like a fruit smoothie or some yogurt will do. However, whether you get up too late to eat, or skip it on purpose, you are doing yourself a disservice by neglecting this important meal. Here is why:

Breakfast literally means "breaking a fast" after a night's sleep. A lot happens when you are sleeping. Your body is in repair mode taking the nutrients you have eaten and using them appropriately for cellular repair and formation, strengthening the immune system, and generally taking care of any messes that were made the day before. When you get up in the morning, you are in a depleted state. Your body needs more nutrition to have the energy and stamina to function throughout the day. If you don't give your body that much needed nutrition, your energy level will be low, your brain cannot function very well, and your metabolic rate stays lower.

Our bodies are like well oiled machines if we give them what they need. Breakfast has a way of kick-starting your metabolism and refueling your depleted energy stores by depositing glucose (sugar) back into your muscles, liver and brain. Without good nutrition after a night of sleep you literally run on empty and if you are a guy, this means taking the fuel from the very muscles you want to build. If you are a girl, you are not saving calories you are depriving yourself of a healthier metabolism which helps you maintain a healthy weight.

Skipping breakfast also contributes to a weakened immune system because you are putting undue stress on all your organ systems by making them try to function without any fuel. Okay, enough said…Just keep in mind that one of the easiest ways to improve your health right now is to have a healthy breakfast of some kind before you get all wrapped up in the day's activities. Oh, and by the way, a strong double latte isn't going to cut it, but we'll chat more about that later.

Breakfast smoothies

Breakfast doesn't mean you have to sit down to a big plate of pancakes, sausage and eggs, in fact it isn't even recommended. For a light but nutrition packed start, try some of these smoothie recipes.

Fruit to go

Serves 1

1/2 cup berries (blueberries, raspberries, blackberries or your favorite)

1/2 frozen banana

1/2 cup milk

1/2 cup orange juice

Blend and go.

Berries

Berries are natural immune system boosters. Anytime you can add them to your diet, you are doing yourself a favor. They are packed with vitamin C and antioxidants that help keep your cells healthy. Berries are also very low in sugar so it's hard to overdo them.

Strawberries

Strawberries are a winner anytime. These nutritionally dense little packages offer more viable vitamin C than even oranges and grapefruit. They are also a great source of potassium and fiber which will help keep your cardiovascular system healthy and strong. Strawberries are also one of the fruits that contain ellagic acid, which may help reduce your risk of cancer. Make sure you buy them organic and if you can't, make sure you wash them thoroughly. For some reason strawberries have one of the highest incidences of pesticide residue so it's important to really get them clean.

Tropical breeze

Serves 1

1/2 cup crushed pineapple

1/2 cup frozen strawberries

1/2 frozen banana

1/2 cup orange juice

1/2 cup milk

1/2 cup plain yogurt, optional

Blend and go.

Pineapple

Pineapple boasts a healthy dose of manganese, a bone strengthening mineral. Just one cup exceeds the daily recommended requirement. In addition, you will get a good amount of copper, thiamin and fiber. The enzyme bromelain helps reduce inflammation in the body also, which is always a good thing.

Since purchasing pineapple can be a gamble at best, here are some tips. Let your nose be your guide. Forget all those other tricks like plucking the middle leaf to check for ripeness. This method is unreliable at best and doesn't guarantee that your pineapple isn't already rotten.

Choose a pineapple that seems heavy for its size. This indicates juiciness and lots of pulp. The leaves should be small and vivid green, not brown or wilted. The eyes should stand out, not be sunken. A ripe pineapple should give a little when pressed. Avoid the one's that feel very hard. Pineapples don't ripen after being picked, they only rot, so pick a good one and eat it as soon as you can.

Bananas

Bananas are so easily digested that they are often the first fruit given to infants. They are also very dense so they are the athlete's choice for a concentrated source of good carbs and potassium before or after a workout. Bananas are also a good source of vitamin B6, a nutrient many people don't get enough of. Vitamin B6 is an important component to keeping your immune system functioning at its peak.

Mango Tango

Serves 1

1 cup milk

1/2 cup orange juice

1 cup fresh or frozen organic mango chunks

1/2 frozen banana

Blend and go.

Mangos

If you have never tried a mango, you don't know what you are missing! The mango is often referred to as the "fruit of India."

When ripe it should be firm and deep shades of yellow, orange, and red. Some will have green in them also and should give a bit to touch. It is common to see a few black spots on the skin but if there are many don't choose it as it is overripe. If the skin is wrinkled it is also past its prime. The skin should be colorful and smooth and it should smell very fragrant.

Mangos are a superior source of vitamin A in the form of beta carotene as are most of the deep orange fruits and veggies. Eating lots of these deep colors is the best way to get your vitamin A. Mangos are also a great source of vitamin C and unlike other fruits, they contribute several B vitamins too. Believe it or not, they also have a good dose of calcium. The peak season for mangos is the warm summer months generally from May through August, June being the absolute best month to enjoy these tropical delights. Here is a tip, if you bring home a mango that is not ripe you can speed up the process by placing it in a paper bag with a ripe mango. Check it frequently as it will ripen extremely fast this way.

Pumpkin spice smoothie

Serves 1

1 cup milk

1/2 frozen banana

1 tsp. pumpkin spice

Blend and go.

Vanilla smoothie

Serves 1

1 cup plain or vanilla yogurt

1 cup milk

1/2 frozen banana

1/2 tsp. vanilla extract

1/2 tsp. Stevia, optional

Blend and go.

Yogurt

If you include dairy products in your diet, yogurt is probably one of your better choices and a good additive to any smoothie. Buying it plain and organic is your best bet nutritionally. It helps boost the calcium and protein content of your shake in a healthier way than some artificially produced powders. Soy yogurt can be a good choice also as it does not contain any cow's milk.

Be careful with protein powders, they often contain all kinds of unwanted additives that do nothing to promote health. Contrary to popular belief, more protein does not translate to more muscle. If you get too much it is just turned to fat like anything else.

Flax

Adding a tablespoon of ground golden flaxseed or flaxseed oil to your smoothie can also significantly boost the nutritional properties of your smoothie. Flaxseeds are rich in omega-3 fatty acids, magnesium, potassium, and fiber. They are also a good source of the B vitamins, protein and zinc. They are low in saturated fat and calories, and contain no cholesterol. They have a nutty taste and can be added to just about anything, liquid or solid, everything from shakes to salads, cereal and soup. Make sure to grind the seeds before adding them as this is how you will benefit from their nutritional value. Adding them whole will most likely get passed right on through your system undigested.

Adding a scoop of Juice Plus+® Complete will also boost the nutritional content of any of these smoothies and can be a good alternative to artificial powders. Check it out!

Eggs & things

Breakfast burritos

Serves 2

2 burrito size whole wheat tortillas

4 eggs or 1 cup egg substitute

2 tsp. butter

2 tbsp. chopped red onion

1 tomato chopped

1/3 cup low-fat cheddar or jack cheese

1/4 cup sour cream, optional

Lightly beat eggs if not using substitute. Melt butter in skillet. Sauté onion and tomato for one minute. Add eggs and scramble until almost set. Add cheese and continue to cook and stir until cheese is melted and eggs are done. Heat tortillas, add 1/2 egg mixture to each tortilla, top with sour cream, fold and eat.

The typical recipe for pancakes can leave you feeling tired, sluggish and ready to chow down again within a couple of hours. This is because they contain too many starchy unproductive carbs. These pancakes will leave you feeling satisfied, energetic and ready to start your day because they have a higher ratio of protein to car~ bohydrate.

Perfect pancakes

Serves 2–3

3/4 cup low-fat cottage cheese

1/2 cup egg substitute or 2 eggs

1/4 cup milk

1/2 cup whole grain flour (more or less depending on how thick you like them)

In a blender combine the cottage cheese, eggs and milk and blend until smooth.

Slowly add flour and blend until thoroughly mixed and desired thickness is achieved.

Pour onto nonstick heated griddle and cook until both sides are light brown, turning them once.

Serve with warm fruit, jam or a little maple syrup.

Blueberry pancakes with spicy blueberry syrup

Serves 4

1 cup whole grain flour

2 tsp. baking powder

3/4 cup skim milk

2 egg whites

1/2 cup blueberries

Combine flour and baking powder in medium bowl. Beat milk and egg whites in small bowl. Add milk mixture to flour mixture stirring until almost smooth. Gently fold in blueberries. Cook on nonstick griddle until golden brown, turning once.

Spicy blueberry syrup

Makes about 3/4 cup

3/4 cup blueberries

1/8 cup maple syrup

1/2 tsp. lemon juice

1/2 tsp. ground cinnamon

1/8 tsp. ground nutmeg

Bring blueberries and syrup to a boil in small saucepan over medium heat. Mash hot berries with a fork. Add lemon juice and spices and stir over medium heat for about 2 minutes. Pour over pancakes.

This egg dish packs a powerful protein punch.

Creamy egg scramble

Serves 4

6 eggs or 1-1/2 cups egg substitute

1/2 cup low-fat cottage cheese

1/4 tsp. dry mustard

1/8 tsp. ground pepper

1/8 tsp. salt

Beat eggs, cottage cheese, mustard and spices until mixed. Pour into nonstick or lightly greased frying pan. Cook stirring constantly until eggs are completely set.

For a variation on this recipe, add 1/4 cup chopped onion, green peppers and tomato to eggs while they are cooking. Use your imagination!

Open faced spanish omelet

Serves 4

This omelet is different from traditional one's in that it is served open faced, not folded.

2 tsp. olive oil

1/2 cup onion, diced

1 cup boiled or leftover potatoes, diced

1/4 tsp. ground pepper

6 eggs or 1-1/2 cup egg substitute

1/2 cup low-fat cheddar cheese

Heat olive oil in large skillet. Add onion and sauté until onion turns transparent. Add potatoes and pepper and continue to cook until edges of potatoes start to turn golden brown. Beat eggs and pour over potato and onion mixture. Sprinkle cheese onto mixture and stir to mix. Cover and cook until egg looks set. With large spatula, turn the entire omelet over and cook until light golden brown.

These soufflés are for the adventurous aspiring chef. There is a bit more work involved but I dare you to give them a try, you just might be the next great chef!

Quick & easy egg soufflé

Serves 6

1 tbsp. butter

1 tbsp. all-purpose flour

1 cup milk

6 eggs, separated

1/2 tsp. salt

Melt butter in a saucepan and stir in the flour. When the mixture is smooth and slightly bubbly, add the milk and continue to cook, stirring constantly, until the mixture has thickened. Remove from heat and allow to cool to room temperature. Beat egg yolks until they are light and lemon colored; add salt; mix well and add to the cooled cream sauce. Beat together until thoroughly mixed. Beat egg whites until peaks form. Gently fold the egg whites into the cream sauce and egg mixture. Pour into a 1-quart, ungreased casserole dish. Place in a 325 degree oven for 10 minutes. Raise the heat to 350 degrees and bake for an additional 15 minutes or until the soufflé is a golden brown and highly puffed up. Serve immediately.

Cheese soufflé

Serves 6

1/4 cup butter

1/4 cup flour

1/4 tsp. salt

1 cup milk

1/2 cup shredded low-fat cheddar cheese

4 eggs, separated

1 tsp. dry mustard

Dash of cayenne pepper

1/4 tsp. ground pepper

1/4 tsp. cream of tartar

Melt butter in saucepan over low heat; stir in the flour and salt and continue to cook over low heat until the mixture bubbles. Add milk slowly and continue to cook, stirring constantly, until the mixture has thickened and coats the spoon. Add shredded cheese and continue to cook and stir until the cheese has completely melted. Remove from heat.

Beat egg yolks until they are lemon colored. Stir 2 tbsp. of the hot cheese sauce into the egg yolks and then add the rest of the yolks to the cheese sauce, mixing thoroughly.

(Failure to do this step may result in the yolks hardening in the hot cheese sauce causing lumps). Add mustard, cayenne, and pepper, and mix again.

Beat egg whites until they begin to get bubbly; add the cream of tartar and continue to beat until stiff peaks form. Gently fold the beaten whites into the cheese mixture, taking care not to over mix which would cause the air to escape from the whites. Pour mixture into an ungreased 1-1/2 quart casserole dish. Place the casserole dish in a pan of water in a 350 degree oven for 1 hour or until the soufflé is puffed up and golden brown. Serve immediately.

Ten tips for a healthier lifestyle

1. **Junk food trashing**: Get rid of all the unhealthy foods in your cupboards and pantry. These will consist mostly of the processed prepackaged foods. Start stocking your frig and cupboards with healthier snack foods such as frozen and fresh fruits, nuts, popcorn, yogurt, low-fat cheeses and veggies you can dip in peanut or almond butter.

2. **Add more fiber**: By adding more fiber to your diet, you can actually block the absorption of other carbohydrates causing a lower carb effect. This is the true way to eat lower carb without all the fancy artificial sweeteners and stuff added in. The best sources of fiber include, whole grains, fruit, beans, legumes and veggies and you should get between 25 and 35 grams per day, minimum.

3. **Make a plan**: Eating healthy can often mean giving it some thought ahead of time. Make a pot of chili or a pot of soup that you can freeze single servings of for occasions when you don't have time to prepare a healthy meal from scratch.

4. **Don't guzzle calories**: Regular soda has over 12 teaspoons of sugar per can and fruit juices tally up almost the same except they do have nutritional value where soda does not. Limit your juice intake to about 1/2 a cup a day and try eating an orange

or some other whole fruit instead. What lacks in juice is the fiber from the fruit it came from which helps slow down the sugar into your bloodstream. Soda is loaded with calories that go down way too easily and often too fast. Diet soda is not a better alternative due to the chemicals it's made from. There is no nutritional value to soda, it can leach calcium from your bones and the artificial sweet-eners they use have been linked to negative health effects.

5. **Add some protein to all your meals**: Adding protein to your meals will minimize blood sugar spikes. Some healthy protein choices include eggs, turkey, lean meat, fish, peanut or other nut butter, chicken, beans, soy or tofu, nuts and low-fat cheeses.

6. **Cut the caffeine**: Although caffeine can give you a feeling of an immediate energy burst, it really isn't energy at all. It is a stimulant that jacks you up temporarily. Although in moderation it can be fine, too much has a way of making you come crashing down just as quick as it picked you up leaving you feeling tired and craving sweets and processed carbs. Here's something you probably didn't know. Too much caffeine triggers the stress response by flooding your system with *cortisol* which is a powerful chemical needed for quick responses and in emergencies. When this happens, your body blocks the ability to burn fat. So, in essence, you are cheat-

ing yourself out of burning fat by substituting caffeine for healthier foods and beverages. It isn't a great diet plan. Moderate amounts vary from person to person depending on individual sensitivity to it. Consuming less rather than more is always a good idea.

7. **Graze**: Rather than eating 3 bigger meals a day, try eating 5 to 6 smaller meals throughout the day. This helps keep your blood sugar level which helps you to avoid getting too hungry and reaching for the wrong foods or eating too much. Plus, you will actually burn calories more efficiently if you don't let your brain think you are starving by getting too hungry. When you are over-hungry, your brain sends a signal to the body telling it to slow down the metabolism since it doesn't know when it will get food again. Our bodies are great at defending themselves. Eating just a little something healthy about every 3 hours is probably a good rule of thumb.

8. **Eat a more plant-based diet**: By eating at least 9 servings of fruits and veggies every day, your body benefits from the phytonutrients found in the various colors in the plants. These, plus the minerals and fiber they contain, help you to fight cancer and disease, and make your cells more sensitive to insulin which helps them function efficiently.

9. **Cut portion sizes**: The number one reason people are gaining weight these days is not only the foods

they are choosing but how much of it they eat. It has been said that we are suffering from what has been referred to as "portion distortion." Use a smaller plate if this is an issue and use your fist as a guide when dishing out portions. Of course, choosing healthier foods allows you to eat larger portions in the first place. A good rule is to have at least 3/4 of your plate filled with plant-based foods and whole grains while the other 1/4 can be a protein or main dish item.

10. **Don't avoid fat**: Fat is not the enemy, the type of fat you consume is. Eating things like nuts, avocados, cold water fish, and olives can help improve the functioning of your brain and heart as well as reduce your craving for sweets and simple carbs because it increases *satiety*, the feeling of being satisfied. Also, getting your healthy fat from food sources rather than adding it to your food in the form of oil is generally a much healthier way to include fat in the diet.

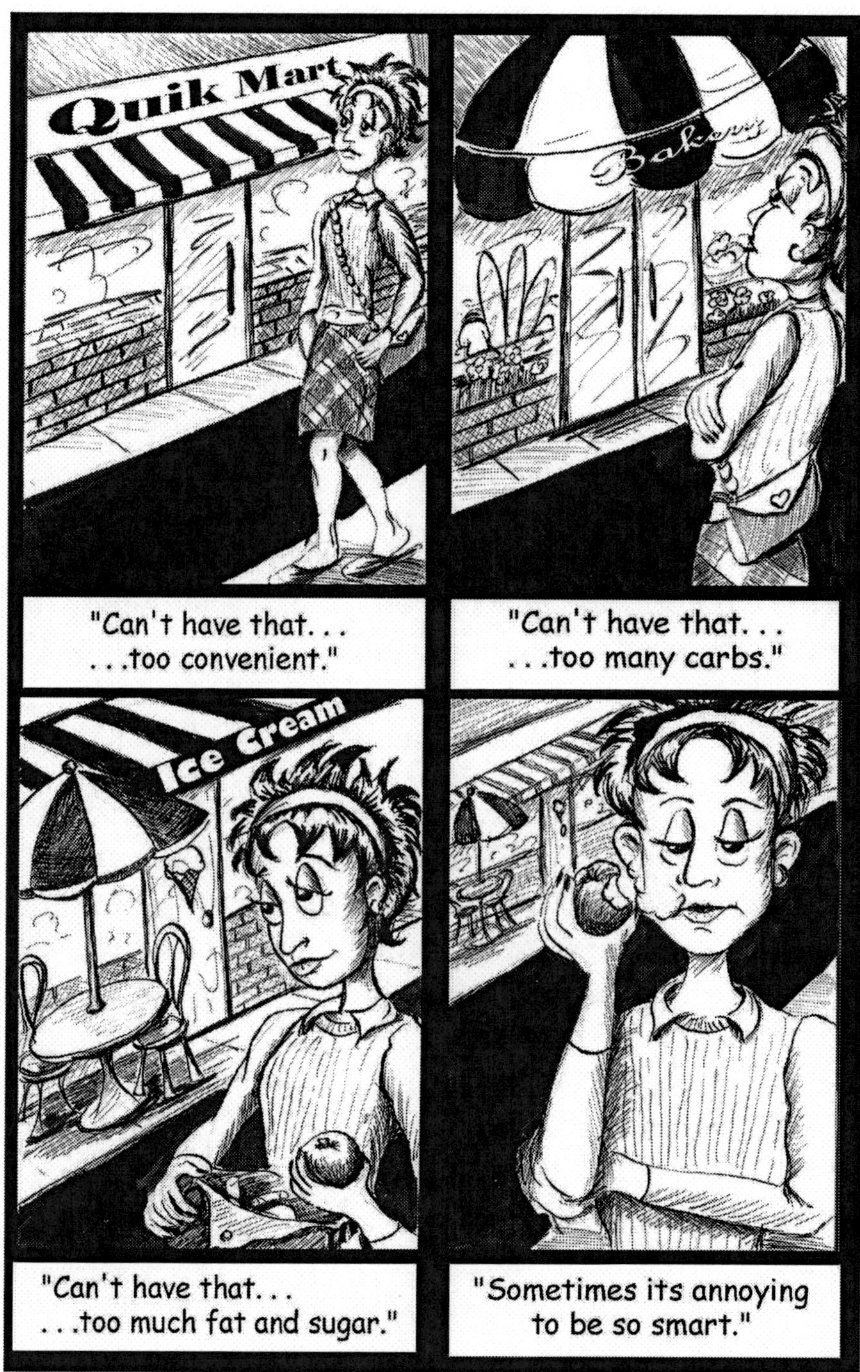

"Can't have that. . .
. . .too convenient."

"Can't have that. . .
. . .too many carbs."

"Can't have that. . .
. . .too much fat and sugar."

"Sometimes its annoying
to be so smart."

Just what is the immune system?

The Immune system is different from the other body systems you are used to. It is not a system of organs nor does it have a single controlling organ. The immune system is comprised of very specific cells scattered throughout your body that have a very specific function. That function is to protect you from foreign invaders. It's kind of like an army of over 200 billion strong marching around your body all the time looking for unwanted intruders to kill like bacteria and viruses. These cells are made in your bone marrow and reside in your lymph nodes, spleen, liver, and *thymus gland* (which is found in your neck a few inches below the thyroid gland) when they are not circulating in your blood.

These cells are your white blood cells and they are very important to you. When you are run down, your army has to work really hard to manage everything that is going on. Sometimes they get bombarded while you are in a weakened state and they get overwhelmed by intruders. That is when you get sick. Your fever is telling you that the war is on between your army and the intruders. Most of the time your army wins the war, but sometimes you have to add doctors and medicine to your artillery to help in the fight. In any case, taking care of yourself, getting good nutrition, exercise, and rest helps your army stay strong so when you need them they can fight for you and win.

Just for girls

Hey girls, feeling a little like your bodies are alien and you can't get out? Yea, I know, we've all been there. In fact, by the time many of you read this, you have probably felt like this from time to time for awhile. The good news is you will grow into your new maturing body and learn how to manage it. The bad news is that yes, you have to go through all stages of the growing and maturing process. Fortunately you have your sister friends to help you through it and they know exactly how you feel. It's important and good to talk with them about it, relate your experiences, your feelings, and how you are coping. Also, your Mom is a great resource, after all she has already been through it.

I wanted to address some of the common issues girls your age face so that you are armed with some insight, know you are not alone, and be able to deal more sanely with them. So, fasten your seatbelts, it could be a bumpy ride!

First of all, it is wonderful to be a woman and you should be proud to be the strong beautiful girls that you are. You all have something special to bring to the world, never forget that. However, there are aspects of your world that may be annoying to say the least.

Do you sometimes feel like you can't control your food cravings?

Are you having more bad hair days than good?

Does your skin break out even though you are using all the products the clear skinned girls on the ads are using?

Do you get moody sometimes for no reason?

Are you gaining weight in places you never did before?

Do you feel bloated and crampy a few days a month?

Well, you are not alone. Millions of girls go through this on a regular basis every month to some degree or another. The main reason for all of these symptoms are hormones. They are what govern all your bodily functions and reactions, help you grow into a woman and at the same time can take you from being a princess one minute, to a raving wicked witch the next without warning.

Female hormones are extremely strong and may sometimes feel out of control. Unfortunately, there is no getting around them, so we have to learn what works for us individually to minimize the symptoms. There is a very delicate balance between the chemicals we produce so when they fluctuate throughout the month they can often wreak havoc on our bodies and mood.

Hormone fluctuation can include some or all of the symptoms I mentioned and there can be varying degrees of discomfort on any given month. Because we are all unique, it is difficult to prescribe any one regimen for everyone. I certainly don't proclaim to know the answers and I am not a doctor so I would never presume to diagnose or recommend any course of action other than to incorporate healthful lifestyle habits to minimize symptoms.

Some girls are very sensitive to changes in hormone levels throughout the month and can practically feel the changes occurring while others seem to skate by. In any case, there are some things you can do to help minimize symptoms.

One of the best ways to tame hormonal symptoms is by cutting down on junk food and sugar. I know, that is generally what we crave, but let's face it, we are what we eat and drink, literally. Our cells are made of the things we put into our bodies. If you give it junk, it's going to fling junk right back at you and that includes contributing to how you feel and handle hormonal swings.

Think about it, have you ever felt crabby after eating a lot of sugar or fast food? How about when you've had a couple of soft drinks with some chips or other salty snack? Come on, a little bloated maybe or irritable? Does your skin and hair sometimes seem too oily or too dry? The way you feel is a direct result of what you have given your body to use as fuel to grow and maintain health (or not). In other words, the brain releases chemicals in response to the kinds of foods we eat. This can determine emotions, mood, and how we look. So, what we eat highly influences whether we will feel good, bad or ugly. Activity level, stress, and rest factor into the equation also.

Now I admit that raging hormones contribute to your moods and emotions but soothing these bad feelings with junk food only causes more of a problem. Imagine if you put soda in your mom's car instead of gas, it wouldn't go very far would it? You get the picture. Having said that, you want to minimize junky carbs like white bread, cookies, chips, fries, etc. These will leave you feeling sluggish and cause you to crave even more carbs. Dairy products are suspected to contribute to acne and various other problems as well. Staying away from caffeine is also a good idea. It can cause food cravings, headaches and irritability.

Some of the best ways I know to minimize symptoms besides eating better is to get enough exercise, water and rest. Exercise can actually reduce cramps in some cases, even though you are less likely to want to get active when you hurt. Exercise releases chemicals into your bloodstream that can often help alleviate pain and elevate mood. Our bodies are truly amazing that way. Our very own body chemicals are stronger and often more effective than drugs. Exercise can also reduce stress and keep your weight down, while rest helps your body heal and regenerate. Try some of the cool yoga and Pilates workouts with your friends. They can help with flexibility, strength and stress also.

Keep in mind that aerobic, strength, and flexibility training go hand in hand. Neither should be emphasized or ignored. Do some of each and you will not only burn

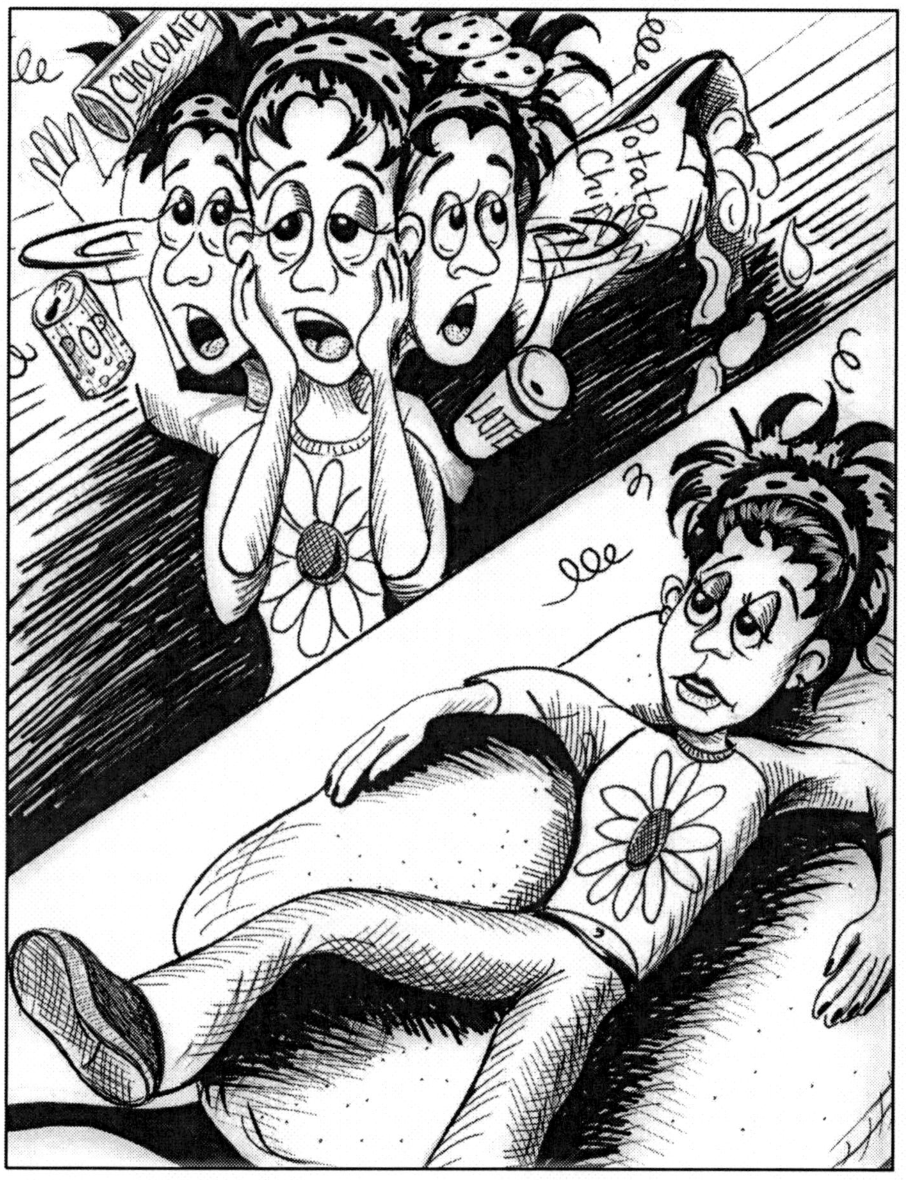

"I need a new personality."

lots of calories, you will have a strong body, toned muscles, and a strong cardiovascular system. Drinking lots of fresh clean water will help flush your system of toxins, alleviate bloat, minimize headaches, help with weight and help clear your skin.

When it comes to skin and hair, buy products that are closest to your natural Ph. Ph is a scale that tells whether something is acidic or alkaline or "basic". Here is how it

Ph Scale

Acidic	0	battery acid
	1	sulfuric acid
	2	lemon juice
	3	soda, orange juice
	4	peroxide
	5	skin, hair, bananas
	6	milk, urine
Neutral	7	pure water
	8	sea water, eggs
	9	baking soda
	10	soap
	11	ammonia
	12	soapy water
	13	bleach
Basic	14	liquid drain cleaner

looks.

Our skin has a Ph factor of about 4.5 to 5.5 If you use a product that is too acidic or alkaline, the natural reaction of the skin and scalp is to return the Ph back to normal. This creates kind of an internal fight within your cell structure which can cause an overreaction of oil or extreme dryness to return the Ph to normal. The one thing you don't want to use on your face is regular bar soap. The Ph is too high and will severely dry out the skin initially.

A good way to tell if you are using the wrong product on your skin is if it feels really tight and dry right after you wash it. More often than not, you will feel oily later which is defeating the purpose and those prone to dryer skin will feel even drier.

Don't know what the Ph of your products are? Every product has a phone number on it for comments or information. Call and ask what the Ph is. If they can't tell you, don't buy it. Good skin care lines will know. Bananas actually have a similar Ph to the skin and make a great facial mask. Also, beware of the acne washes and scrubs. They are notorious for stripping your skin of all its natural moisture and protective *acid mantle*, causing a rebound effect which will often result in more oiliness and more blemishes caused by bacteria invasion.

The *acid mantle* is actually just a fancy way of describing the layer of protective oils and sweat secretions that help kill germs on the top layer of your skin and protect your skin from bacteria invasion. So stripping it off with harsh scrubs, alcohol and other astringents leaves your face vulnerable for a few hours while your Ph is trying to rebalance itself. It's like removing a protective shield. Also, it's not a good idea to scrub your face especially if it is broken out, you will just spread the infection. It will also stimulate the oil glands in your skin causing even more oiliness. Be gentle and kind and it will be more gentle and kind back.

It is also important to use a good moisturizer even if you think you have oily skin. Contrary to what you might think, moisturizing will not cause your skin to be more oily. In fact, by giving your skin moisture, you help to suppress the body's reaction to release more oil. Many people find that they really don't have oily skin at all, they are just not treating it correctly. But, if you are truly prone to blemishes and oily skin, there are gentle and effective cleansers and moisturizers that are formulated specifically for that skin type. Using the same product line from cleanser to moisturizer is also helpful since the ingredients are formulated to work *synergistically* together. Synergistic means working in harmony with each other. Using several different brands of products at a time can cause confusion within your cells while they try to figure out what you are trying to achieve. It really is all about chemistry.

So, I can't promise that all your symptoms will magically disappear by following this advice, but I'm willing to bet that you will feel better more of the time.

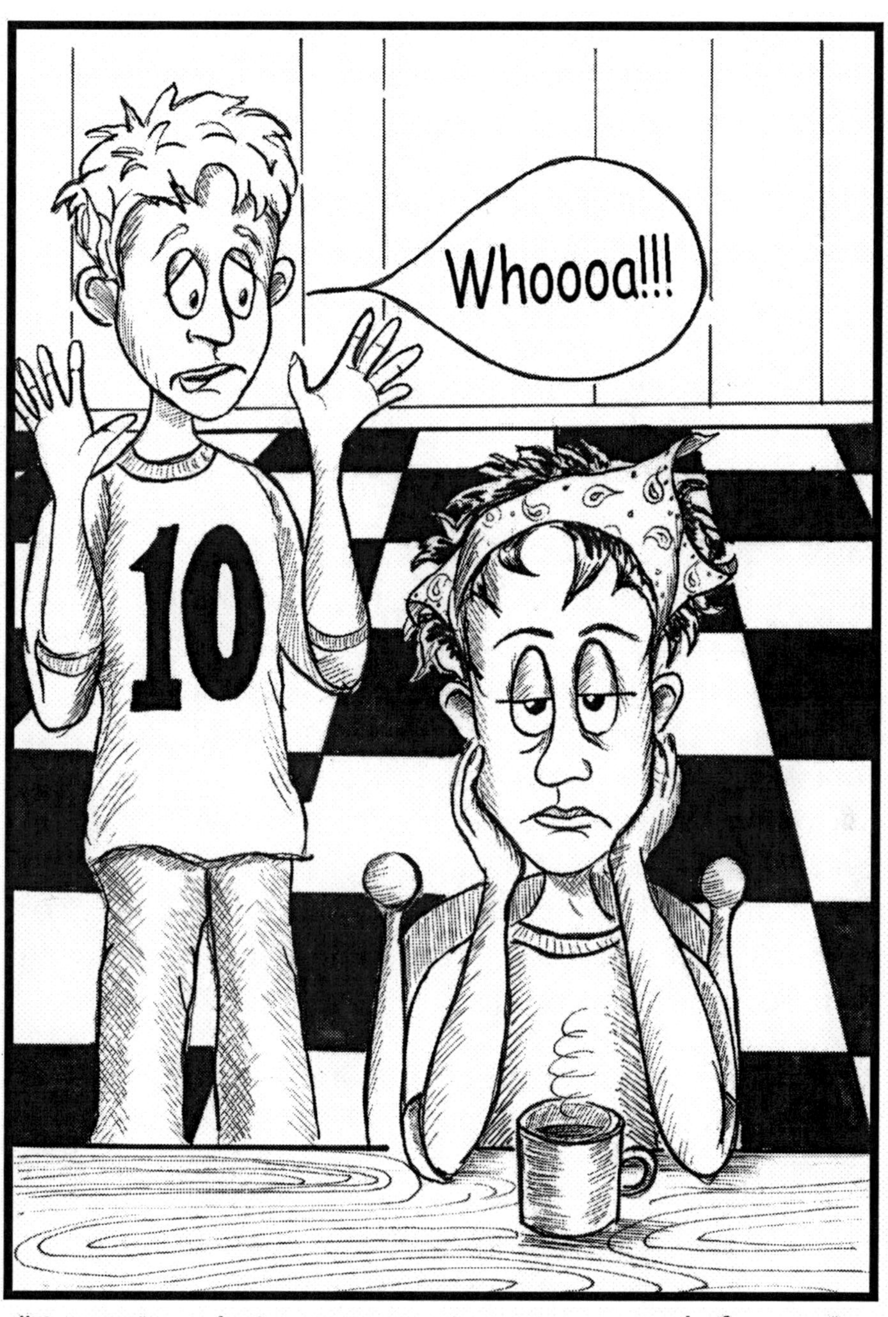

"Sometimes being a woman is just too much for me."

Now, what about that pesky weight gain? Unfortunately, once puberty hits, gaining some weight is common and Mother Nature's way of transforming you from a girl to a woman. It doesn't happen to all girls, heredity plays a small role in all that too. Our bodies have a wonderful way of ensuring that our species survives. Sometimes, women who are dangerously thin have a hard time conceiving a baby. Being too thin can cause hormone production to be too low and without the proper balance, things don't always function correctly. So, it's a delicate balancing act all the time.

Also, if a girl exercises so much that her fat stores go below a certain threshold, the normal female hormone balance can get out of whack also and sometimes cause menses to stop. This is not a healthy state to be in as hormones are very important to lots of normal bodily functions and the maturation process. If left untreated for long periods of time, negative consequences could occur that might not show up until later in life. It's so important to pay attention to what is going on with your body. It's a good idea to discuss some of these issues with your doctor if they ever become a concern.

Let's talk a bit more about the importance of exercise since most of us probably won't fall in the category of exercising too much.

The closest thing to a magic bullet for maintaining your youth and optimal health is a well balanced combination of exercise and good nutrition. The entire body benefits from this formula. Regular exercise improves digestion and elimination, increases endurance and energy, promotes lean body mass while burning fat, helps lower weight and stress levels, and improves overall mood.

So, while good nutrition is fundamental to a healthier you, it is only part of the equation. A regular exercise routine is optimal but not always realistic due to hectic schedules and school work. One of the things you can control on a regular basis though is your general activity level throughout the day. For example, park farther away from the stores at the mall so you get an extra walk. Take the stairs instead of an escalator or elevator. Help out with the household chores. Take your dog for a walk. Take a walk around the block while you talk to your friends on your cell phone. Wash the family car. Ride a stationary bike while you watch your favorite TV show. You get the idea. The more active you are all day, the more calories you will burn all day too. Of course adding a regular exercise program to your week or participating in school sports activities are great ways to stay fit. And, adding some of these other activities on a regular basis will certainly help.

Why so much emphasis on exercise and good nutrition? Not only does it help you stay lean and fit, it can help you stay healthy as you get older. Sometimes there can be a tendency toward developing a certain disease because of your family history. But, whether you develop it may depend on how you live your life. Living an unhealthy lifestyle can take its toll and tip the scales in the wrong direction. You may not have control over your heredity but you do have control over how you live and the choices you make every day. Remember junk in equals junk out. Not everything is inevitable, your choices may very well tip the scales in your favor. The odds are definitely worth it.

The truth about artificial sweeteners

The problem with sugar is that it doesn't have any nutrients so when you consume too much you crowd out room for healthier foods. On the other side of that coin you have artificial sweeteners which are getting more and more negative press as adverse health effects begin to emerge. These sweeteners really should be avoided if at all possible. If you can use fruit, juice or *Stevia* to sweeten things, these are better choices. Stevia is a natural sweetener that comes from a plant. You can generally find it in whole or health food stores. Maple syrup and honey can be used in very small amounts also as an alternative to table sugar. Apple sauce makes a great sweetener and can even substitute for extra oil in your baking recipes. You will notice that most of the recipes in this book use it instead and you won't notice a difference in taste only in nutritional and calorie value.

What's the big deal? Well, decades ago it was found that some artificial sweeteners could possibly cause cancer and were taken out of products and off the shelves. In response to needing an alternative, a new substitute was manufactured. The FDA said it was the recommended alternative and put it in all sugar free products. Some people, women in particular, have experienced negative side effects as a result of ingesting it in their usual products. Later it was found that due to a chemical reaction in the body, it can act as a neurotoxin (one that affects the brain and nervous system). It is now speculated to contribute to mimicking symptoms of Alzheimer's, MS, Parkinson's, and a host of other neurological diseases. While it hasn't been taken off the market as of yet, we should all be wary.

Again in response, another sweetener is out and its claim to fame is that it is a healthy alternative to other artificial sweeteners because it is made from sugar. Yes, it is manufactured from sugar molecules but in order for it to be converted to the artificial sweetener manufacturers have to use a process whereby they chlorinate it. Hello, I said chlorinate! We know chlorine is a known *carcinogen* (cancer causing agent) and shouldn't be consumed in any amount, and since we don't know how the chemical structure will affect people in the long term it might be best to err on the side of caution and not become the guinea pig for such a study. The bottom line is that we should cut down on sugar, but subbing chemicals for it is probably defeating the purpose. I don't know about you, but I'm not willing to use my body as a test tube, are you?

And then there are *sugar alcohols*. Sugar alcohol usually ends in "tol" on labels. These can be an okay alternative in very small amounts as they do not affect blood sugar as much as the real thing, but too much can cause gastric distress, bloating, cramps and diarrhea. You will find sugar alcohol in many of the new low carb candies and chocolates on the market today as well as foods that are acceptable for diabetics. It is important to read the label and pay attention to portion size. This is one time when not heeding portion size can have some not so pleasant side effects. It is good that diabetics and those sensitive to sugar have an alternative, but keeping foods that contain sugar and sugar alcohol to a minimum is your best bet since the foods that contain them are not the most nutrient dense and healthiest choices to begin with.

Breads & muffins

Apple cinnamon muffins

Makes 12

21/4 cup oat bran

1/4 cup brown sugar

2 tsp. cinnamon

1 tbsp. baking powder

2 tbsp. vegetable oil

1/2 cup nonfat milk

3/4 cup apple sauce

2 egg whites

1 medium apple, chopped

1/2 cup walnuts, chopped

1/4 cup raisins, optional

Mix dry ingredients in large bowl. Mix oil, milk, apple sauce, and egg whites in a bowl. Add to dry ingredients and mix. Add chopped apple, nuts, and raisins. Fill lightly greased muffin tins and bake in 425 degree oven for 17–20 minutes.

Corn bread

Makes 12 servings

1 cup yellow corn meal

1 cup whole grain pastry flour

1 tbsp. baking powder

1/2 tsp. salt

3/4 cup nonfat milk

1 egg

2 egg whites

3 tbsp. butter, melted

Preheat oven to 425 degrees. Combine dry ingredients. Add milk, egg, egg whites, and butter. Stir to mix. Pour into 9x9 inch lightly greased baking pan. Bake for 20–25 minutes. Serve warm.

Lunch stuff

Pita pizza

Serves 1–2

1/4 cup pizza sauce

1/3 cup shredded mozzarella cheese

1/4 cup chopped onion

1/4 cup chopped bell pepper

1 whole wheat pita

Spread pizza sauce over top of pita. Sprinkle cheese, onion and bell pepper on top of sauce. Place 4 inches below heat source in broiler until cheese is melted and veggies look cooked.

If you don't like bell peppers and onions, use any other fruit or veggie toppings you like.

Quesadilla

Serves 1

1 whole wheat tortilla

1/4 cup low-fat cheddar or jack cheese

1 tomato diced

1/4 cup onion, diced

Sprinkle all ingredients over half the tortilla and fold. Heat in microwave for 30 to 60 seconds or for a crispier texture, heat on nonstick griddle until cheese is melted, turning once. Top with salsa, avocado, or sour cream if desired.

Tuna salad sandwich

Serves 1–2

Tuna is a good source of lean protein that also contains healthy omega-3 fatty acids. Tuna can contain some mercury depending on where it was caught much like some other large ocean fish like swordfish and albacore although chunk light tuna contains less. It is also a good idea to only choose dolphin safe tuna when you do buy it.

1 3oz. can water packed solid white albacore tuna

2 tbsp. low-fat mayo or nonfat yogurt

1 tbsp. raisins

1 tbsp. celery, minced

1 tbsp. apples, minced

1 tsp. mustard

Pepper to taste

1 whole grain pita

1/2 cup sprouts or chopped dark green leafy lettuce

Combine first 7 ingredients. Cut pita in half and stuff tuna mixture equally into both halves. Add 1/4 cup sprouts or lettuce on each half.

Egg salad sandwich

Serves 4

7 hard boiled, free range eggs

1/2 cup diced celery

1/3 cup sweet pickle relish

1/2 tsp. salt

1 tsp. mustard

1/4 tsp. ground pepper

3 tbsp. of your favorite mayo

8 slices whole grain bread

Lettuce or sprouts

Slice eggs in half and take out 3 yolks, put them aside. In a medium bowl chop the rest of the eggs into small pieces. Add celery, relish, salt mustard, and pepper. In a small bowl, take the 3 yolks and mash them with a fork. Add mayo and mix until creamy. Mix the dressing with the egg mixture. Spread on bread with lettuce or sprouts.

Why choose organic & natural?

When it comes to meat, poultry, eggs and dairy products, there really isn't a choice if you want the best for your health and you want to include these in your diet. Not every ranch can have the organic designation as it can be pretty difficult to get. There are quite a few variables that need to be considered. However, if the label says "natural" there are rules that determine that status as well and they are preferred over animal products that cannot claim this on their labels.

When your product says *certified organic* it generally means that the animals have been raised to graze freely in their natural habitat and eat the food that is natural to them in a non-crowded environment. This helps keep the animals healthy and less stressed. This means a healthier and more natural product for you. These products will probably cost a bit more but completely worth it. Research the companies you buy from though, as some of them may use different standards that may not be as optimal.

It is just as important to buy organic produce. They do make a huge impact on health. When pesticides are used, it is not always possible to wash them all off. In fact, some fruits and veggies are more prone than others to pesticide concentration. Strawberries and basil tend to keep more pesticide residue on them, while produce like carrots and other root or tubular veggies may have the ability to absorb more pesticides causing higher concentrations on those vegetables. (Here's Health, 1996) For these reasons alone, you should seek out organically and naturally grown produce and animal products whenever possible.

Ten super foods you should eat

1. **Whole grain/high fiber Bread**

    Fiber helps to balance the carbohydrates and since the grain is in its whole natural form, it has all the original vitamins and fiber in it that has not been removed and refortified like white flour has.

2. **Cantaloupe**

    1 quarter of a cantaloupe supplies almost as much vitamin A and C as most people need in an entire day.

3. **Broccoli**

    You simply cannot get a larger dose of nutrients than by eating broccoli. Not only is it a great source of vitamins C and A (mostly in the form of beta-carotene) but it also comes with healthy doses of folic acid, fiber and believe it or not, calcium. For those who don't eat many foods naturally high in calcium, broccoli offers a very absorbable dose. Calcium is an important component to keeping bones healthy and strong. It's best to get calcium from foods over supplements as the body doesn't recognize isolated calcium as well as it does from a food source.

4.   **Sweet potatoes**

This is a nutritional all star and one of the most nutritious vegetables you can eat. They are loaded with carotenoids, vitamin C, potassium, and fiber.

5.   **Watermelon**

Excellent source of vitamin C and carotenoids, low in calories and tastes great on a hot summer day.

6.   **Beans**

Inexpensive, versatile, low in fat, rich in protein, iron, folic acid and fiber. Great choices include gar-banzo, pinto, black, Navy, and kidney beans.

7.   **Salmon and other fatty fish**

The omega3 fats in fish, especially fatty fish like salmon, sardines, mackerel and rainbow trout can help reduce the risk of cardiovascular disease.

8. 100% bran cereal

A half cup serving of this cereal provides about 1/3 of the fiber you need for an entire day. Moving food waste products out of your system faster helps reduce the risk of cancer and other diseases.

9. Strawberries

These sweet little treats are high in vitamin C, potassium, fiber, antioxidants, and are low on the sugar reaction scale and low in calories.

10. Spinach and kale

Loaded with vitamin C, carotenoids, calcium and fiber. Also very beneficial to eye health and helps reduce risk of cancer.

Eleven foods you should avoid!

1. Potato chips

Regular chips are deep fried in over heated cook-ing oils. These rancid fats wreak all kinds of havoc in your body possibly setting you up for some major grief down the road if these are a staple in your diet. Oh, and stay away from the fat free vari-ety unless you really want stomach cramps and

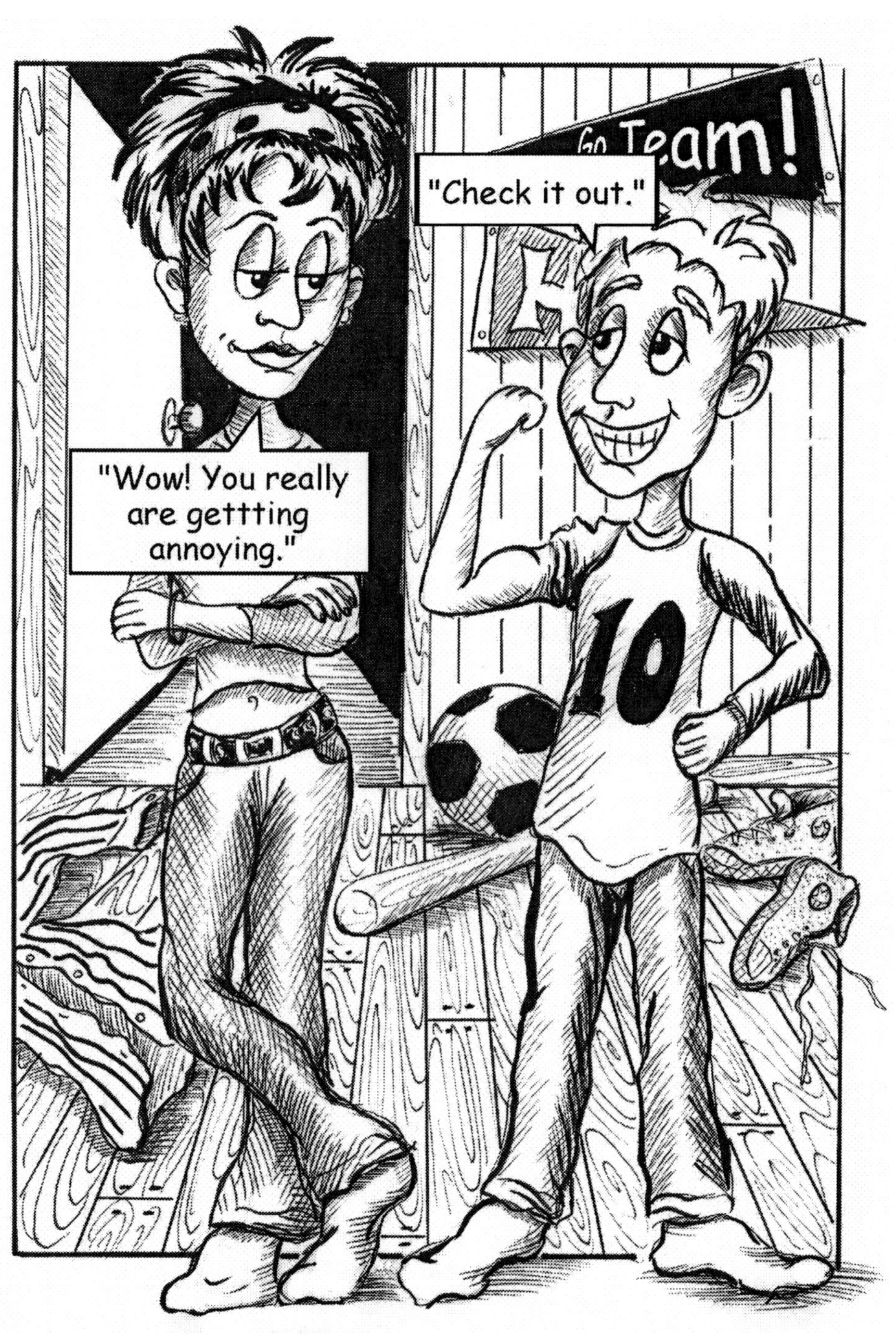

Go Team!
"Check it out."
"Wow! You really are gettting annoying."
10

diarrhea. The artificial fat they fry these in isn't
recognized by the body so it will definitely let you
know it's not happy! Also, because of the chemical
structure of the fake fat they use in these, many of
the vitamins and minerals you are eating with the
chips pass right on through your system without
being absorbed. So, if you must have them, try
some of the baked varieties, they are not fried,
don't contain trans fat, and have less calories. Be
aware though, researchers have just discovered a
chemical called acrylamide in many chips, regular
and baked, that could contribute to cancer and
other problems. The research on this is ongoing, so
go easy, we don't clearly know the ramifications of
this discovery. Plus, eating too many crowds out
room for healthier foods.

2.   Prepackaged alfredo sauce

Talk about a heart attack on a plate! There is so
much fat in this sauce you may as well melt a stick
of butter on your pasta and call it good. Try the
recipe in this book for Alfredo sauce, I'll bet you
don't even miss all that fat.

3.   Double or over-stuffed pizza

Simply having 2 slices of this cheese pizza will put
you over the edge when it comes to salt (2200mg)

calories (800) and saturated fat (17g) which could
put you over your total daily intake recommendation. This is all before adding any pepperoni or
sausage. Anytime a restaurant boasts that their
pizza weighs in over 3 pounds before baking is a
hint to try something else. Thin crust pizza can
actually be a pretty healthy choice once in awhile
as long as you keep portion size under control, put
some veggies on it, and couple it with a healthy
salad.

4. Frosted doughnuts

How can one doughnut have as much artery clogging saturated and trans fat (10 grams) as nine
strips of bacon? That's what happens when you
cover a doughnut completely with frosting. Dough-
nuts are never your healthiest choice but if you
must have one, try some of the plain baked ones on
the market today.

5. Prepackaged oriental noodle soups

The noodles are prefried in artery clogging palm
oil. A serving of this soup looks like a traffic jam to
your arteries, not to mention the salt content of
those unassuming little packets of spices they come
with. Try 1,020mg in one serving. That's almost
half your daily allowance. If you like these, try
some of the healthier brands you can get at most

whole food stores or make your own using organic
chicken broth and whole wheat pasta skipping the
flavor packet in favor of some of your favorite
spices and herbs.

6.   Regular canned soups

A small can of soup can contain your entire
allowance of salt. The label might say it has about
1,100 mg per serving. There are generally at least 2
servings per can so you do the math. Who sits
down to a half a can of soup anyway? You can find
healthier alternatives if you look, but your best
choice is to make it yourself. Try some of the
recipes in this book, I'll bet you even like them better.

7.   Sandwich cookies

Can you say junk? Talk about artificial, I'm not
sure there is anything natural in these. The
prepackaged cookie is bad enough, but then fill it
with a sugary concoction of fat and chemicals and
all I can say is yuck! Cookies are not something
many of us want to give up on totally so make your
own. At least you will know what's in them.

8.   Regular granola

Do you think Mother Nature intended for you to
get your oats covered in sugar and laden with
more artery clogging fat that a fast food burger? I

think not! If you are stuck on granola, at least buy the low-fat version and keep your portion size to a minimum. Better yet, use it as a topping on a healthier cereal like oatmeal or shredded wheat. You'll still get the flavor, just not all the fat, sugar and calories.

9. French fries

These are probably the absolute worst thing you can put in your mouth. That's why I've saved them for last. They are probably one of the biggest reasons today why there is so much obesity and heart disease on this planet. They've taken a perfectly good vegetable and turned it into the most salty concoction of rancid fat you can get. Potatoes lend themselves to soaking up as much of that over-heated oil as possible, making every bite one nail closer to the coffin. Sorry, sad but true. They also don't break down over time so what happens to them inside your body? Ever found one under your car seat or couch like a year later and it looked and smelled the same as the day you bought it? Hello…

Everyone loves them though so try making your own, there is no comparison on the health scale and I'll bet if you give them a chance you won't even miss the others. There's a recipe right in this book for a healthier version, go on give them a try.

10. Margarine

Margarine was one of those brilliant inventions that came about because it was thought that butter was an unhealthy choice. Since people wanted to spread some sort of fat on things, science came up with the artificial version. For years it was believed to be safe and a good alternative. After a few more decades of research scientists have discovered that not only is it a very unhealthy choice it is merely one molecule away from being plastic! Yea, I want that in my body. At least our bodies know how to digest butter, used sparingly of course. And, to be fair, there are a few healthier butter substitutes out there now made from olive oil and that contain plant phenols. Do your homework if you want to try them, and use them and butter very sparingly.

11. Onion rings

Do I really need to go there?

If you leave a regular fast food burger in its styrofoam container and put it on a shelf in the garage, it will still look the same as the day you put it in there a year later. Yummy!

Ten more super foods

1. **Oranges**

    Wonderful and especially good during the winter months when they are at their peak of flavor. Attributes include vitamin C, folic acid, and fiber.

2. **Blueberries**

    Blueberries are one of those wonderful fruits nature provided for us to help brain function and eye health. They contain properties that help with blood pressure, cholesterol, and cardiovascular dis-ease. They are also really low on the sugar reaction scale so eat up.

3. **Apples**

    They say an apple a day keeps the doctor away and they may be right. There are over 10,000 phytonu-tients in a fresh ripe apple. Apples are great for your digestion and actually act as a scrubber for your lower intestine, helping to keep that organ system healthy and you running smooth. They are high in fiber and low on the sugar reaction scale. Apples are one of the foods that actually burn more calories eating them than they contain.

4. **Garlic**

    Raw garlic has a reputation for helping arteries stay clear of clots and may help lower cholesterol.

The National Cancer Institute is conducting studies on garlic's ability to fight certain cancer. In any case, garlic is a wonderful flavor enhancer and probably has more health benefits than we have discovered yet.

5. Tofu/soy

If you like to eat on the lighter side, tofu and other soy products contain a good source of vegetarian protein and are a good source of calcium. One of tofu's best qualities is its ability to take on the flavors of whatever you are cooking it with. It has a mild flavor on its own and is a great additive to smoothies and soups as well.

6. Nuts

Nuts are another great way to get heart healthy fat in your diet. They are high in calories so you need to eat them sparingly, but, they are a wonderful protein and mineral source. Believe it or not, the peanut, which is actually not a true nut but in the legume family, has the most complete protein. Nuts are a good complement to grains and other vegetables boosting nutritional value.

7. Papaya

If you want to find a really nutrient-dense fruit, this is it. Papaya boasts two very important antioxidant nutrients, vitamins A and C. These two vitamins when consumed by eating the foods containing them have shown promise in reducing risk of cancer, heart disease, and *cataracts*. Cataracts are growths on the eye that can impair vision. And papaya's generous potassium content can help keep blood pressure in check.

8. Avocados

Avocados are actually considered a fruit and as fruits go they are pretty high in calories and fat although there is benefit to the fat in avocado since it is monounsaturated, the same type found in olive oil, which is great for your heart and skin. We do need some fat in our diets and avocados are a great way to incorporate healthy fat in the diet.

9. Onions

Like garlic, onions seem to have similar health benefits. They are believed to have anti-cancer and cholesterol lowering properties as well as help to prevent blood clots. Here again is a chance to flavor your food with this potent bulb over salt. And if you like green onions, the green stems offer a good dose of vitamin A.

10. Bananas

The athlete's choice for quick energy. It is a great pre-workout food since it is easily digestable and easy on the digestive system. It's also a great alter-

native to other potential snack foods. It has a high
potassium content which helps keep blood fluids
balanced as well as help to keep blood sugar more
stable.

Snacks

Quick & easy vegetable dip

Makes 2 cups

2 cups fat-free sour cream

1 pkt. Ranch dressing mix

Mix packet into sour cream and chill. Serve with raw veggies of your choice.

Wise chips

Serves 1–2

2 burrito size whole wheat tortillas
Salt and/or cayenne to taste

With scissors, cut tortillas into triangles, chip size. Sprinkle just a tiny bit of water over tortillas so that seasoning will stick. Sprinkle seasoning on tortillas. Bake on baking sheet at 450 degrees for 12 minutes or until crisp. Serve with salsa.

Fresh fruit fondue with creamy lime dipping sauce

Makes 12 servings

Use any fruit you like with this dip. The following ingredients are just suggestions.

2 tbsp. lime juice

1 small jicama, peeled, cut into cubes

1 lb. watermelon, cubed, rind removed

1 small pineapple, peeled and cubed

2 ripe papayas, seeded, peeled and cubed

10 strawberries

1 cantaloupe or honeydew melon, cubed, rind removed

Sprinkle lime juice over jicama so it doesn't brown. Arrange fruit on a plate. Serve with lime dipping sauce.

Lime dipping sauce

Makes 2 cups

12 oz. nonfat vanilla yogurt

4 tbsp. minced fresh cilantro

4 tbsp. lime juice

1 tbsp. minced jalapeno pepper

1 tsp. sugar

Combine all ingredients and mix well. Refrigerate until ready to use.

Get the fondue forks out and enjoy with friends!

Potato crisps

Makes about 1 cup

1 raw potato, with skin

1 egg white, whipped

Seasoning of choice

Slice potato into 1/8 inch rounds. Brush egg whites over potatoes with basting brush. Season with salt and pepper, cayenne or a little lime juice. Bake at 350 degrees for 20 minutes, turning once.

Even a better alternative here is to use sweet potatoes over white. Sweet potatoes are highly underrated. They are packed with good stuff like beta carotene, vitamins B, C and fiber. They have a wonderful natural sweetness to them and yet they provide less of a sugar reaction than a regular potato. Try them, you might just love them!

Veggies with herb dip

Serves 2–4

Sliced veggies of choice

Slice up your favorite veggies such as carrots, celery, radishes, broccoli, sweet peppers etc.

Dip:

Makes 1 cup

1 cup low-fat cottage cheese

2 tbsp. chopped onion

1 tsp. Italian herb seasoning

1/2 tsp. cayenne pepper

Mix and refrigerate. Dip veggies for a nutritious snack break.

Nachos

Serves 4

*These nachos combine beans, corn and cheese to create
a complete protein equal to that in meat but without all
the fat.*

1 cup chopped onion

1 tbsp. chili powder

2 tsp. dried oregano

2 tbsp. water

1 can (15oz) pinto or black beans, rinsed
and drained

2 tomatoes, chopped

3/4 cup shredded low-fat jack or cheddar
cheese

3/4 cup frozen corn, thawed and drained

1/4 cup sliced black olives

1/4 cup jalapeno slices, drained

Lightly grease medium saucepan. Over medium heat
sauté onion until it is transparent, about 5 minutes. Add
chili powder and oregano and cook for 1 minute. add
beans and 2 tbsp. water and mash with fork or potato

masher until blended yet chunky. Return to heat and cook
6–8 minutes. Set aside.

Make smart chips:

8 corn tortillas

Ground red pepper

Sprinkle tortillas with a little water just to dampen. Shake
off excess water. Cut into wedges, chip size. Sprinkle with
red pepper. Arrange on baking sheet and bake 4 minutes
at 375 degrees, rotate baking sheet and bake an
additional 2–4 minutes. Do not let them get brown. Cool.

Arrange chips on platter or large plate. Sprinkle cheese
evenly over chips. Spoon beans over chips. Spoon corn
and tomatoes over beans. Bake again for 8 minutes or
until cheese is melted. Top with olives and jalapenos.
Serve with salsa and low-fat sour cream if desired.

So what about vegetarian diets?

Many teens are turning toward the trend of a more vegetarian diet. Whether this is a fad or an aim at a healthier lifestyle, caution needs to be heeded since being a true vegetarian isn't just a matter of not eating meat. It takes education in order to get the proper combination of nutrients to maintain good health and nutrition. One of the primary problems of an uninformed attempt at vegetarianism is the tendency to eat too much fat in the form of cheese, dairy products, breads, fried vegetables, and French fries as well as other junk carbs. Many end up gaining weight and being malnourished at the same time. Simply taking meat out of the equation does not a vegetarian make.

Since meat and other animal products can provide the most readily available source of iron and complete protein, vegetarians need to make a special effort to combine their plant foods correctly in order to maximize their nutritional value. Combining legumes, beans, grains, leafy greens, and dried fruits properly can make it work but, it does take education and some work to have a balanced diet. Those that are true vegetarians and know how to combine their foods can be some of the healthiest people on the planet and there is definitely something to be said for going that route, but only if you do it right.

The cost of not practicing vegetarianism correctly is

nutrition imbalance, anemia, calcium deficiency, and a lack of many other important nutrients. If you are interested in a vegetarian diet, it is smart to visit with a qualified nutrition professional such as a nutritionist or dietitian for a comprehensive plan. The key is seeking out a qualified professional. Some people call themselves nutritionists when in reality they have no educational background in the subject. Ask for credentials and educational background before paying money for advice.

I cannot emphasize this point enough. If you are seriously contemplating a dietary change like vegetarianism, make sure to do your homework as well as seek the advice of a registered dietitian or certified nutritionist before starting such a program. They can help you plan your meals and show you how to live a vegetarian lifestyle correctly.

Salads

Anyone can make a green salad. That's why you will find that these are all a little off the beaten path. Salads should be fun so go ahead, be adventurous and give these a try.

Caribbean delight

Serves 4

1 cup plain nonfat yogurt

1 tbsp. vanilla extract

2 tbsp. orange juice concentrate

1 cup brown rice, cooked

1/2 cup canned, crushed pineapple

1 banana, chopped

4 oz. mandarin orange sections

1/2 cup toasted slivered almonds

In large mixing bowl, combine yogurt, vanilla and orange juice; mix well. Add remaining ingredients and toss.

Yellow, red &
green chopped salad

Serves 4

2 cups frozen corn, thawed

3/4 cup tomatoes, chopped

1/2 cup cucumbers, chopped

1/4 cup green peppers, chopped

1/4 cup red onion, chopped

Mix all ingredients in large bowl.

Dressing:

3 tbsp. rice wine vinegar

2 tsp. olive oil

1/8 tsp. salt

Dash pepper

Mix dressing ingredients in container with lid. Shake
well, pour over salad and toss to mix thoroughly.

Spring vegetable pasta salad

Serves 4

3 cups whole wheat spiral pasta, cooked

1-1/2 cups broccoli florets

1/2 cup carrots, sliced

1-1/2 cup zucchini, sliced

2 to 3 free range, skinless chicken breasts

Dressing

3/4 cup nonfat yogurt

1/4 cup apple cider vinegar

2 tbsp. parmesan cheese

2 tbsp. lite mayonnaise

1/2 tsp. garlic powder

1/2 tsp. ground black pepper

Bake chicken breasts 30 to 40 minutes until done and no longer pink inside. Cool and dice. In a small bowl, mix yogurt, vinegar, parmesan, mayo, and seasonings. Set aside. In large bowl, combine pasta, vegetables, yogurt mixture and chicken. Mix well and chill thoroughly before serving.

The "not in the mood for a salad" salad kabob

Serves as many as you want to make

Combine any of the following ingredients and put on skewers for a nutritious and fun way to eat a salad:

Cucumber, avocado, cherry tomatoes, olives, green pepper, onion, carrots, celery, pineapple, apples, zucchini, etc. Alternate veggies on skewers for maximum visual appeal.

Dip in your favorite dressing and enjoy!

Tuna & avocado salad

Serves 2

Avocados are a nutritional winner. Avocados are actually classified as a tropical fruit rather than a vegetable. They supply a healthy dose of monounsaturated fat and ounce for ounce, avocados provide 60% more potassium than a banana and have more beta carotene than most other fruits. Believe it or not, they also contain a healthy dose of fiber. And, they taste great in just about everything.

1 large avocado

1 sm. can albacore tuna packed in water, drained

1–2 tbsp. spicy or wasabi mayo

1 tsp. lemon juice

1/4 cup diced red onion

1/4 cup diced celery

1 tbsp. pickle relish, optional

4 lg. lettuce leaves

Slice avocado in half lengthwise and remove pit and skin.

Mix tuna with mayo, lemon juice, onion, celery and relish. Spoon half of tuna mixture into each avocado half. Arrange lettuce leaves on plates. Place tuna stuffed avocado halves on lettuce leaves and enjoy.

85

Bueno mexican salad

Serves 8

1 large red pepper, diced

1 can (15 oz.) black beans, rinsed and drained

1 can (15 oz.) pinto beans, rinsed and drained

1 cup whole kernel corn

1 can (4oz.) diced green chilies

2 green onions, thinly sliced

1/2 cup diced tomato

1/2 cup shredded cheddar or jalapeno jack cheese

8 large lettuce leaves

8 corn tortillas

Mix first 8 ingredients together in a bowl. Add dressing below and toss. Spoon 8 equal portions of salad onto large lettuce leaves. Serve with warm corn tortillas.

Dressing:

1 tbsp. white wine or cider vinegar

1 tbsp. rice wine vinegar

2 tbsp. lemon juice

1 clove garlic, minced

1 tbsp. olive oil

1/2 tsp. ground cumin

Combine all ingredients in small bowl; mix well. Pour over salad just before serving.

What is a carotenoid anyway?

Carotenoids are a class of phytochemicals, *phyto* meaning plant. They are essentially fat soluble pigments found in yellow, red, green, and orange vegetables and fruits. The darker the produce the more carotenoids they contain. They are a potent family of antioxidants that help keep our cells healthy and strong to prevent disease. Of the more than 500 found in nature, about 50 of them can be converted into vitamin A in the body. The neat thing is that when you get *beta carotene* (one of the carotenoids that converts to vitamin A) from foods, the body knows just how much to convert to vitamin A depending on how much you need. The left over continues to act as an antioxidant to help prevent cellular damage from things like sunlight and air pollution. Since none of it goes to waste there is no chance for toxic build up in our bodies *unlike taking an individual vitamin A or beta carotene supplement in the high dosages they come in.* In fact, recent studies suggest that taking 50,000 international units or more daily in supplement form may interfere with normal cell division. Just another reason to stick with how Mother Nature intended us to get it (Balch & Balch, Prescription for nutritional healing, 2000).

So then what is an antioxidant?

Antioxidants are substances that protect the cells in your

body from *oxidation.* You get them from eating fruits and vegetables and other healthy food sources as mentioned above. Oxidation is a natural chemical process whereby oxygen molecules react with other molecules in the body to create destroyer compounds called *free radicals.* Just as the student radicals of the 1960's liked to stir up trouble, free radicals try to wage a war against your healthy cells. Some examples of oxidation are when you cut an apple and it turns brown or when milk and butter go rancid, or your car rusts. This process all starts with oxygen. Interestingly, if you put lemon juice on a cut apple it doesn't turn brown. That is because the vitamin C in the lemon juice acts as an antioxidant to prevent the oxygen from doing its damage. Get it?

Oxygen is a bad thing?

Obviously we need oxygen to live and breathe. If we didn't have it, we would cease to exist on this planet. I know it seems to be a double-edged sword that the very oxygen we need can harm us. Our bodies are naturally equipped to deal with this oxidation process which is a natural part of living, however, poor eating habits, environmental pollutants, and too much stress have made it difficult to keep everything in balance. These lifestyle factors tend to increase the amount of oxidation that occurs in the body. This is why we need to be more aware of what we eat. In order for our bodies to keep up with the fight, we need the ammunition. Eating a healthier diet is a great way to keep those antioxidants in your arsenal.

And a free radical is?

Free radicals are the destroyer compounds that result from the chemical process whereby oxygen molecules react with other molecules causing negative effects. This is what is known as oxidation. They are not foreign invaders though, they are a normal result of metabolism that are produced by the millions through every day activities as well as from things like environmental pollutants and UV. It's complicated, but they are a sort of by-product of living in general, just as smoke is a result of a fire burning.

Our bodies have a built in protection mechanism that can protect itself from the damaging chain reactions that free radicals can set off. However, if we do not get enough antioxidants in our diets, free radicals can get out of control and out pace our body's natural repair system. Some of the more harmful culprits that contribute to this are bad food choices, cigarette smoke, ultraviolet light from sun exposure, and environmental pollutants such as smog, car exhaust, ozone, and household chemicals. Left unchecked, these free radicals can damage healthy cells to the point of actually altering the genetic make-up of normal cells in the body. Once these cells start dividing abnormally they can cause all kinds of problems like cancer, tumors and disease. Antioxidants help prevent all of this damage by neutralizing free radicals before they can do their harm. So, getting enough antioxidants from the foods we eat is sort of like rust proofing our bodies (Webb & Smith, Foods for Better Health, 1995).

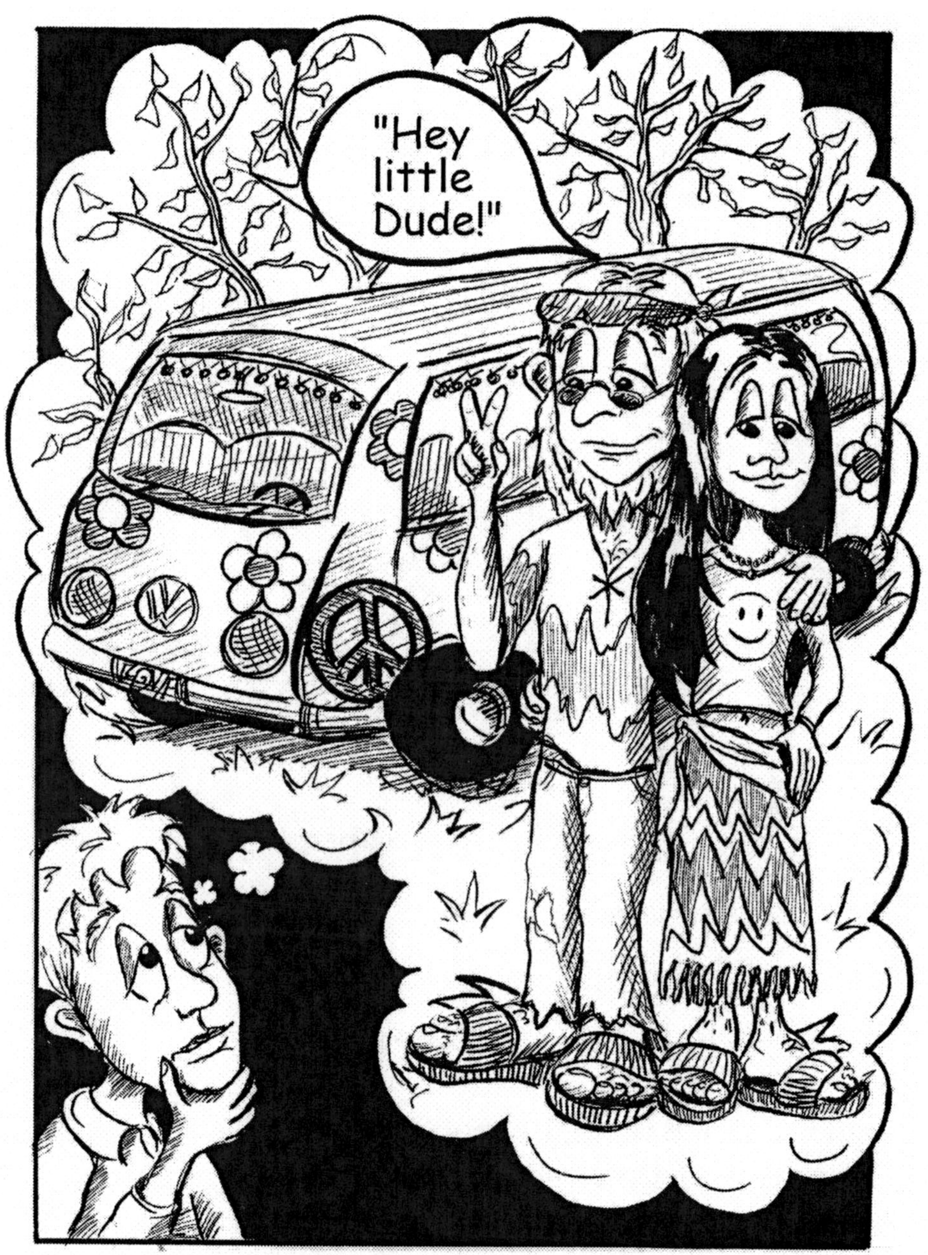

"... and I thought free radicals were those guys back in the 60's with the big flowers and peace signs all over their Volkswagon buses.

Soups

Simple minestrone

Serves 6–8

1 quart water

1 (10oz) pkg. frozen mixed veggies, your choice

3 oz. uncooked whole grain pasta, whatever you like

2 chicken bouillon cubes or 2 tsp. granules

1/2 tsp. dried basil

1/2 tsp. dried oregano

1/2 lb. sliced fresh mushrooms

2 carrots, sliced

2 zucchini, sliced

1 (15 oz.) can diced tomatoes

Combine first 6 ingredients in stock pot or Dutch oven; bring to a boil. Cover, reduce heat, and simmer 5 minutes. Add mushrooms, carrots, zucchini, and tomato; stir well. Cover and cook an additional 20 minutes or until carrots are crisp tender.

Fresh tomato soup

Makes 4 cups

1 tsp. butter

2 tbsp. shallots

3 cups tomatoes (2 lbs) peeled, seeded and diced

3/4 cup low-fat milk

1/2 cup low sodium chicken broth

1/2 tsp. salt

Dash white pepper

Fresh oregano leaves, optional

Melt butter in large saucepan over medium heat; add shallots. Cover and cook 5 minutes or until tender. Add tomatoes, cover and cook 15 minutes. Place tomato mixture in blender, add milk, broth, salt and pepper. Cover and whirl 5 seconds. Return tomato mixture to saucepan and cook over medium heat 5 minutes or until heated. Garnish with fresh oregano leaves, if desired.

Corn chowder

Serves 4

1 tsp. olive oil

1/2 cup celery, diced

1/2 cup onion, diced

1/4 cup green or red bell pepper, chopped

2 cups fresh corn kernels or 1 (10oz.) pkg.
frozen corn

1 cup potatoes, diced

1 tbsp. fresh parsley, chopped or 1 tsp. dried

1 cup low sodium chicken broth

1/2 tsp. paprika

1/8 tsp. white pepper

2 tbsp. unbleached flour

1/2 cup low-fat milk

1-1/2 cup nonfat evaporated milk

Heat olive oil in a large saucepan. Sauté celery, onion and
bell pepper until soft. Add corn, potatoes, parsley, broth,
paprika and pepper. Bring to a boil, then simmer for
10–15 minutes or until potatoes are tender. In a jar with
a tightly fitting lid, combine flour and 1/2 cup milk.

Shake to blend thoroughly. Slowly add to chowder stirring constantly. Add evaporated milk. Cook and stir over medium heat until mixture thickens. Serve with crusty whole grain bread.

Easy tex-mex beef soup

Serves 4

1/2 lb. boneless grass fed beef round steak,
cut into 1/2 inch cubes

1 tbsp. olive oil

1 cup onion, chopped

1 clove garlic, minced

2 cups water

1 (15 oz.) can diced tomatoes

1 cup carrots, chopped

1 (8 oz.) can kidney beans, drained

1/2 cup green bell pepper, chopped

2 vegetable or beef bouillon cubes

2 tbsp. tomato paste

1 tbsp. chili powder

1 tsp. cayenne pepper

1/4 tsp. pepper

In large saucepan, cook beef, onion and garlic in oil on
medium heat until meat is brown. Stir in the remaining
ingredients. Cover and simmer about 30 minutes or until
meat is tender.

Chunky chicken noodle soup

Serves 4–6

1 lb. boneless, skinless, free range chicken breasts

1qt. water

3 fresh celery leaves

3/4 tsp. poultry seasoning

1/4 tsp. dried thyme

2 cups water

2 cups whole wheat broad noodles, uncooked

1/2 cup sliced celery

1/2 cup sliced carrots

1/3 cup green onion, sliced

2 tbsp. fresh parsley, minced

2 tsp. vegetable or chicken bouillon granules

1/2 tsp. black pepper

Combine chicken, 1 quart water, celery leaves, poultry seasoning, and thyme in a large stock pot; bring to a boil. Cover, reduce heat and simmer 45 minutes or until chicken is tender. Remove chicken from broth, reserving broth. Let chicken cool. Coarsely chop chicken and add back to broth. Combine chicken and broth with the 2 cups water, and remaining ingredients in large stockpot; bring to a boil. Reduce heat, and simmer an additional 25 minutes, stirring occasionally until noodles are done. Serve.

Creamy carrot soup

Serves 4

2 tbsp. butter

2 tbsp. light cream cheese

6 carrots, sliced

1 onion, chopped

1 clove garlic, crushed

2 medium potatoes, diced

5 cups organic chicken broth

1 cup low-fat sour cream or plain yogurt

In large saucepan melt butter and cream cheese. Add carrots, onion, and garlic and cook for 3 minutes. Stir in potatoes; reduce heat to low. Cover and cook for 15 minutes. Add chicken broth and purée soup in blender until smooth. Pour back into saucepan and heat through. Stir in sour cream or yogurt and stir until bubbly. Serve.

What is cholesterol?

When we hear about cholesterol we generally think of it as a bad thing. In actuality, we need cholesterol in order to produce the various hormones that we need to function normally. It is also an essential component of every cell in our body. This is why our livers make the majority of the cholesterol that we have. We can also get cholesterol from the foods we eat. However, we can only get dietary cholesterol from animal foods like dairy, eggs, cheese, and meat products. We cannot get it from vegetables and nuts because these things do not have livers and we now know that the liver is what produces cholesterol.

Now there are some other things that are believed to contribute to bad cholesterol levels such as "hydrogenated" vegetable oils, trans fats, smoking etc. Consequently we want to limit our exposure to these negative things. Just keep in mind that the only foods that actually contain cholesterol are animal foods because they have livers that produce it. There is a difference between factors that contribute to blood cholesterol levels and the foods we consume that actually contain it. Vegetables and nuts do not have livers so they cannot produce cholesterol but some can contribute to cholesterol levels which will be discussed further. I know I said that twice but there seems to be confusion about this when we read labels so I thought it was important to reiterate.

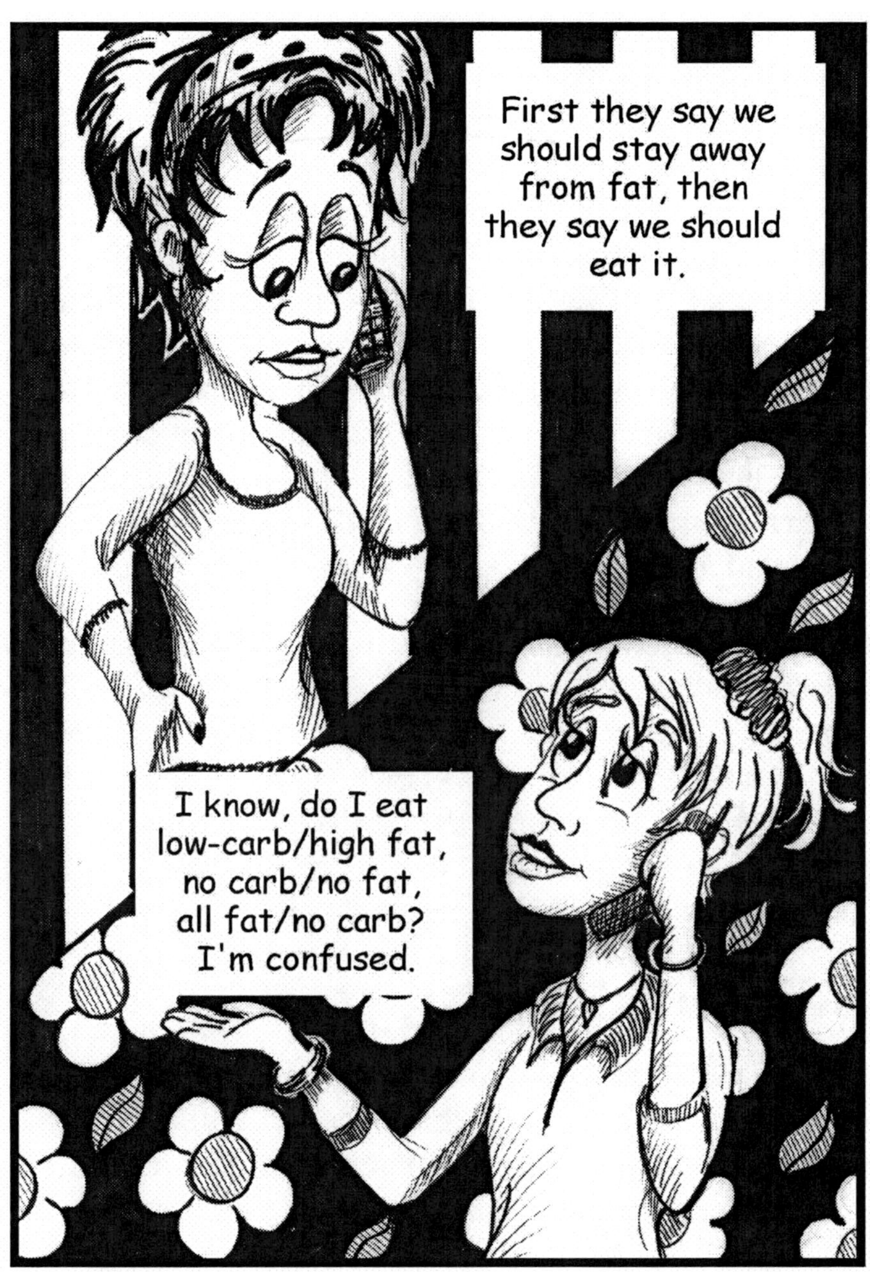

First they say we should stay away from fat, then they say we should eat it.

I know, do I eat low-carb/high fat, no carb/no fat, all fat/no carb? I'm confused.

The two most talked about types of cholesterol are HDL and LDL. The way you can remember the difference is by referring to HDL as "healthy" and the LDL as "lousy". The HDL cholesterol goes around the bloodstream mopping up LDL cholesterol and transports it back to the liver where the liver disposes of it, while the LDL cholesterol comes out of the liver and tries to attach itself throughout your arteries potentially causing problems. So, it is good to have enough good cholesterol to control the bad. It's essentially a matter of balance. There are some other factors involved, but you can do a lot to help by eating healthy and staying away from foods you know are high in the bad stuff.

Be careful of some of the marketing ploys products like vegetable oil and peanut butter use. They will say "no cholesterol" right on the label. Don't be fooled into paying more for these, you already know that they are cholesterol free by nature. However, if the label says it contains partially hydrogenated oil it can contribute to bad cholesterol, but we will discuss that next.

Demystifying Fats

With all the publicity surrounding fat, it's confusing to say the least. After reading this page, you will be armed with information about the differences and be able to make better choices for good health.

There are several types of dietary fat.

These include:

Saturated

Polyunsaturated

Monounsaturated

Omega-3 's

Hydrogenated (trans fat)

First let me give you some of the benefits of including fat in your diet. Good fats in the diet help enhance the absorption of some nutrients and transport fat soluble vitamins, help promote hormone production, and support growth. It is good for your skin and hair and it provides a concentrated source of calories that helps you feel satisfied when you eat. Typically, people who eat a high carb, very low-fat diet tend to not feel as satisfied, which often can result in over-consumption and binging on the wrong foods.

Good fats come primarily from plants, nuts, seeds, avocados, some fish and meat sources. These include omega-3's, monounsaturated and polyunsaturated fats. Monounsaturated fats are the best for heart and cardiovascular health. Good examples of where these can be found are almonds, cashews, peanuts, pecans, avocados, nut oils, grapeseed, canola and olive oils. Including these in small amounts helps reduce the LDL or "lousy" cholesterol. They also help promote the rise in HDL, the good or "healthy" cholesterol. About 10% of your total calories should come from these types of fats and it is always better to get them from food rather than adding oil to get them.

Omega-3 fatty acids are also very heart healthy and are found primarily in flaxseed, pumpkin seeds, walnuts, soy beans, tuna, cod, mackerel, salmon, and halibut.

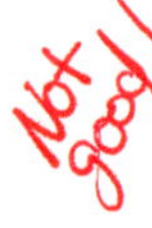

Polyunsaturated fat also comes mostly from plants, nuts and seeds and oils that come from corn, sunflower, safflower, cottonseed, and sesame. These oils have their place in our diets but should be restricted to less than 10% of your total calorie intake as these can lower total cholesterol meaning both the good and the bad. Our goal is to keep good cholesterol high so choose these sparingly.

Then there are the not so good for you types. Saturated fats are primarily found in animal products such as milk, cream, eggs, butter, cheese, meat, and poultry. They are generally those that are solid at room temperature. Some vegetable products contain saturated fat as well such as coconut, palm kernel oil, and shortening which can contribute to bad cholesterol as well. The liver uses saturated fat to manufacture cholesterol. Therefore, excess consumption of these fats tends to raise the bad cholesterol in the blood. It can also lower good cholesterol leaving us vulnerable to heart and cardiovascular disease. These fats should be very minimal in the diet and consist of less than 7% of total calories consumed. Optimally your total fat intake should be around 20% of total calories consumed, not to exceed 25% maximum.

The worst threat to health are trans fats. These fats have been artificially manufactured. These first started showing up about 20 years ago to prolong the shelf life of processed foods. They are abundantly found in prepackaged baked goods such as crackers, pastries and cookies and of course deep fried products like chips and fries. Over 65% of prepackaged foods have some trans fat. The real danger about trans fat is that the body does not recognize what it is and doesn't know how to process it, digest and eliminate it. So, it sticks to artery walls and coats our cell membranes making it harder for the body's cells to communicate and function as they should with each other. Some have likened it to adding a coating of Teflon over our cell membranes. Having read about the eleven foods that should be avoided earlier in this book we know that margarine is chemically only one molecule away from being plastic. Yikes!

The FDA has determined that there is zero tolerance for trans fats in our diet so limiting and even eliminating them from our diets as much as possible is very important. Labels are just now starting to add trans fat content to the list of ingredients of certain foods. By 2006 all prepackaged items will have to include it. The easiest way to know whether something has trans fat in it is to check the label for "partially hydrogenated" or "hydrogenated vegetable oil". It's not good enough to see zero grams next to trans fats on labels. The government allows one-half gram per serving to be counted as "zero". If you eat more than one serving, you are getting trans fats. You can avoid them with a little diligence. For example, choose only nut butters that have the oil floating on top and don't include "hydrogenated" oils on the label. If it is smooth and consistent looking it most likely has trans fat. Making food at home rather than buying it prepackaged is also a great way to limit your exposure and have some control. Trans fats are responsible for many of the health problems we are facing today and must be taken more seriously.

When good fats go bad

Fats and oils are very vulnerable to exposure to air, sunlight, and heat. Overheating (to smoking point) damages the molecular structure and literally renders it a bad fat for your arteries and cells. For some reason vegetable oils are particularly vulnerable. How do you tell if it has gone bad? Smell mostly. Any product that contains fat such as crackers, nuts and peanut butter can go bad if not stored properly or kept too long. When in doubt, throw it out. Eating it may not make you sick like food that is contaminated by bacteria, but rancid fats contain chemicals that can damage cells, maybe even contribute to cancer and clogged arteries.

Okay, so now you no longer have to wonder what is what in the world of fats and cholesterol. Information has the power to change your health in very significant ways. Put that knowledge to practice and you'll be amazed at how good you can feel.

Fat in our diet is essential and shouldn't be avoided completely, but, it is always better to get it from healthy food sources rather than adding it during cooking. The exception to this is when you have salad or a vegetable dish that doesn't have any fat in it at all. Then it can be a good idea to add just a touch of a good fat like olive or grapeseed oil to make the nutrients in these foods more readily absorbable since many vitamins in veggies are *fat soluble*. This means that they need a little fat with them for transport to be absorbed optimally into our systems. Remember that a little goes a long way, use it sparingly, and avoid cooking with it when possible.

Sides

Believe it or not, the eggplant is a close relative to the potato. Though it isn't high in any one nutrient, it is low in fat and very filling, making it a good main dish vegetable. Typically, eggplant is dark purple, but there are also white varieties. It is a native of India. It was not known to Europeans until the twelfth century when Arab traders introduced it to Spain. For some reason in Europe, it got the reputation for causing madness, not to mention leprosy, cancer and bad breath, which prompted its use as a decorative plant. But, by the eighteenth century it was established as a food in Italy and France. It is very versatile, however, it has the ability to absorb more fat than any other vegetable including potatoes, so it's important not to cook it with too much fat, otherwise, you will get all the calories from the fat you use to cook it with.

Baked eggplant & tomatoes

Serves 4

1 small unpeeled eggplant, thinly sliced

1 tsp. salt

3 medium tomatoes, thinly sliced

2 tbsp. dried basil or 1/3 cup fresh, chopped

3 cloves garlic, minced

1/3cup grated parmesan cheese

Place eggplant slices in a colander and sprinkle with salt. Let sweat for 30 minutes. Drain well and pat dry on paper towels. In a lightly buttered 8x8x2 inch baking dish alternately layer eggplant, tomatoes, garlic, basil, and cheese. Cover and bake in a 400 degree oven for 30 minutes. Uncover, baste with baking juices. Bake uncovered for 15 minutes more or until brown.

Note: If mixture appears to be too dry during baking, add a little chicken broth as needed.

Spicy broiled bananas

Serves 4

This one is very unusual and reserved for the adventurous cook!

2 bananas

1 tsp. butter, melted

1 tbsp. minced onion

1 tbsp. lime juice

2 tsp. brown sugar

1 tsp. minced jalapeno pepper

Cut bananas lengthwise into halves, leaving peels on the banana halves. Brush cut sides of bananas with butter. Combine onion, lime juice, sugar and jalapeno in small bowl; mix well. Sprinkle cut side of bananas with onion mixture. Place bananas on rack of broiler pan. Place pan 4 inches from heat. Broil 2 to 3 minutes or until topping bubbles and bananas are heated through. Serve with scrambled eggs or French toast or as an unusual side dish at dinner.

Zucchini schooners

Serves 4

4 medium zucchini

1/2 cup ricotta cheese

1 tsp. Italian seasoning

1 clove garlic, minced

1/4 cup bread crumbs

2 tbsp. parmesan cheese

Cut zucchini in half lengthwise. Steam until tender (about 3 minutes). Scoop out inside of zucchini leaving the shell. Place the zucchini pulp in a bowl and mash with fork. Mix in ricotta, Italian seasoning, and garlic and mix well. Stuff zucchini shells evenly; sprinkle bread crumbs and parmesan cheese over top. Place under broiler for a few minutes until cheese and bread crumbs are browned.

Homemade refried beans

Serves 6

1 cup dried pinto beans (about 6 oz.)

4 cups water

1 cup onion, chopped

1 tsp. garlic minced

1/4 tsp. salt

1/2 tsp. ground cumin

Soak beans overnight in water just enough to cover. Drain beans and place in heavy saucepan with 4 cups water, onions, garlic, salt and cumin. Bring to a boil; reduce heat and simmer 2 hours until beans are soft enough to mash. Mash with fork or blend beans in a blender to desired consistency.

Creamy garlic mashed potatoes

Serves 6

1-1/2 lbs. Idaho potatoes, peeled and quartered

4 cloves garlic, peeled

2 tsp. butter

1/2 cup milk

1/4 cup low-fat sour cream

1 tsp. salt

1/2 tsp white pepper

Bring large saucepan of water to a boil over high heat. Add potatoes and garlic, reduce heat and boil gently, uncovered for about 20 minutes or until potatoes are tender. Transfer potatoes and garlic to large bowl. Add butter and coarsely mash potatoes and garlic with potato masher or fork. Make a well and pour in milk and sour cream. Using a hand mixer, beat the mixture until light and creamy. Add salt and pepper while mixing. If necessary add a bit more milk to achieve a creamy texture.

Guiltless french fries

Serves 4

4 potatoes, washed and left unpeeled

2 egg whites, beaten

Salt or your favorite seasoning to taste

Cut each potato in half around the middle. Using a knife or apple corer, cut potatoes into slices. Arrange potato slices on nonstick baking sheet. Using a basting brush, brush egg white over tops of potatoes. Sprinkle, salt, garlic salt, cayenne or whatever you like lightly over top. Bake in preheated 400 degree oven for about 35 to 45 minutes until golden brown and crispy, turning once after about 20 minutes.

Most people love macaroni and cheese. However, the problem with traditional macaroni and cheese is that many of us eat too much in one sitting. This makes for a very unbalanced meal of too much fat and too many carbs with no fiber. A prescription for weight gain if eaten often.

I also specifically put this recipe under "sides" rather than main dishes even though it is a healthier version of the original because I believe that we should enjoy this dish in small portions. This way, it doesn't have to exit completely out of the diet and be dubbed a "bad" food choice. Although, you shouldn't eat this too often. Remember variety creates balance.

Enlightened mac & cheese

Serves 6

8 ounces uncooked whole wheat elbow mac~aroni

1 tbsp. all-purpose flour

2 tsp. corn starch

1/4 tsp. dry mustard powder

1 can (12 oz) evaporated skim milk

1 cup shredded reduced fat medium sharp cheddar cheese

1/2 cup shredded reduced fat Monterey Jack cheese

1 tsp. Worcestershire sauce

1/4 tsp. ground black pepper

2 tbsp. bread crumbs

Preheat oven to 375 degrees. Cook pasta according to package directions, omitting salt. Drain and set aside. Combine flour, cornstarch and mustard in medium saucepan; stir in milk until smooth. Cook over medium heat, stirring occasionally, until slightly thickened. Remove from heat; stir in cheeses, Worcestershire sauce and pepper. Add pasta; mix well.

Lightly grease 1-1/2 quart casserole dish with butter. Spoon mixture into casserole; sprinkle with bread crumbs and bake 20 minutes or until bubbly and heated through.

Fettuccini alfredo on the light side

Serves 6–8

2 tbsp. butter

1–2 tbsp. garlic powder

1–2 tbsp. flour

1-1/3 cup milk

2 tbsp. cream cheese

1 cup freshly grated parmesan cheese

4 cups cooked fettuccini

Melt butter in saucepan over medium heat. Add garlic powder; stir until smooth. Stir in flour with whisk. Gradually add milk, stirring with whisk until blended. Cook until thickened and bubbly, stirring constantly to make sure there are no lumps remaining. Stir in cream cheese. Cook about 2 minutes until cheese is melted. Add parmesan cheese stirring constantly until melted and a smooth consistency is reached. Toss with pasta, add pepper to taste.

Crunchy chicken nuggets

Serves 4

2-1/2 cups cornflakes

1/2 cup parmesan cheese

1/2 tsp. salt

1/2 tsp. onion powder

1/4 tsp. garlic powder

1/8 tsp. pepper

1 lb. boneless, skinless, free range chicken breast strips

1/4 cup flour

1/2 cup egg substitute

Preheat oven to 425 degrees. Coat baking sheet with nonstick cooking spray or preferably use a nonstick baking sheet. Crush cornflakes in resealable plastic bag with rolling pin or heel of your hand. Pour into shallow bowl. Add parmesan, salt, onion powder, garlic powder, and pepper. Coat chicken in flour. Dip into egg mixture. Roll chicken in cornflake mixture. Arrange chicken in single later on baking sheet and bake 12–15 minutes until golden brown; Dip into your favorite sauce.

Just what is a carbohydrate?

The much maligned carbohydrate is actually the primary way we fuel our bodies and brains. It can be likened to high octane fuel if we choose the right ones. Most experts believe we need about 60% to 65% of our diet to come from carbohydrates in order to have adequate amounts of energy available to get through our active lives. Believe it or not, *glucose* is the only fuel our brains want to convert to energy. Glucose is the result of breaking down the carbohydrates we eat into a highly absorbable form of sugar our cells can use.

There are primarily two types of carbohydrates, *simple and complex*. Simple carbs are generally those that are easily passed into the bloodstream but not necessarily in a healthy way. Simple carbs or simple sugars as they are sometimes referred to, are those that come from things like juice, cookies, cakes, pies, candy, white bread, white rice, and pasta etc.

The problem with sugar is that it doesn't have any nutrients so when you consume too much you crowd out room for healthier foods.

It is important to minimize these types of foods in our diets. Since they get into the bloodstream quickly they can give us a quick sugar rush which then causes a "crashing" effect soon after. Some people experience a "sugar hangover" headache after eating simple carbs. The reason is that when sugar gets into the bloodstream quickly it stimulates the secretion of *insulin*. Insulin is the hormone that regulates blood sugar level and is made in the pancreas. Such a sudden boost in insulin can cause blood sugar to drop just as suddenly as it tries to move the sugar out of the blood, leaving you feeling weak or tired and craving more sweets. Plus, all this high insulin response can cause weight gain as well as wear out the insulin pump. The combination of too much sugar in the diet in the form of sweets and simple carbs and being overweight is contributing to the high incidence of diabetes and other conditions in kids and adults today.

Eating lots of simple carbs also causes a vicious cycle of eating more and more of them as your blood sugar yoyo's up and down. Some people feel they are addicted to carbs and in some ways they are right. The good news is that if you take these "white" and sugary foods out of your diet or at least keep them to a minimum you can kick the habit and stop the yo-yoing affect, not to mention be healthier.

What is less known is that whenever you eat a high sugar content food you can suppress your immune system for several hours afterwards leaving you susceptible to infections or colds and viruses. It is better to limit your intake of these types of carbs. They are the primary culprits of carbohydrate's bad rep. A good rule of thumb is to try and stay away from white foods, minimize sugary foods and reach for the whole grains instead.

The other type of carbohydrates are complex

carbohydrates. Complex carbohydrates by nature have more fiber. They generally come in whole grains, beans, legumes, and in fruits and veggies. Fiber is a key component because it will slow the absorption of sugar into the bloodstream giving you a more healthy sustained energy and a lower insulin response. This keeps your blood sugar more even. Our bodies need these carbs for good health but in reasonable portions. As mentioned previously 60% to 65% of total calories is a good percentage to shoot for and much of that percentage should come from fruits and veggies over breads, cereals or pasta. The good news is that if you choose carbs that are high in fiber you are automatically eating lower carb because for every gram of fiber that is in the food you can deduct one of the carbohydrate grams. Here is one example. There are high fiber tortillas on the market today that boast up to 21 grams of fiber! You heard me right, by eating only one of these burrito size tortillas you get over half your day's worth of fiber. So if there are 34 grams of total carbohydrates in the high fiber tortilla you really only have to count 13 since you can subtract 21 grams because of the fiber. These 13 carbs are called *net carbs* because they are the one's that will contribute to your total intake. Compare that to a regular "white" tortilla which has the same number of carbs but only 1 gram of fiber. Obviously it is best to get most of your complex carbs and fiber from fruits and veggies but as you can see, this one small change can make a big difference, cool huh?

I used this example because it was pretty extreme and

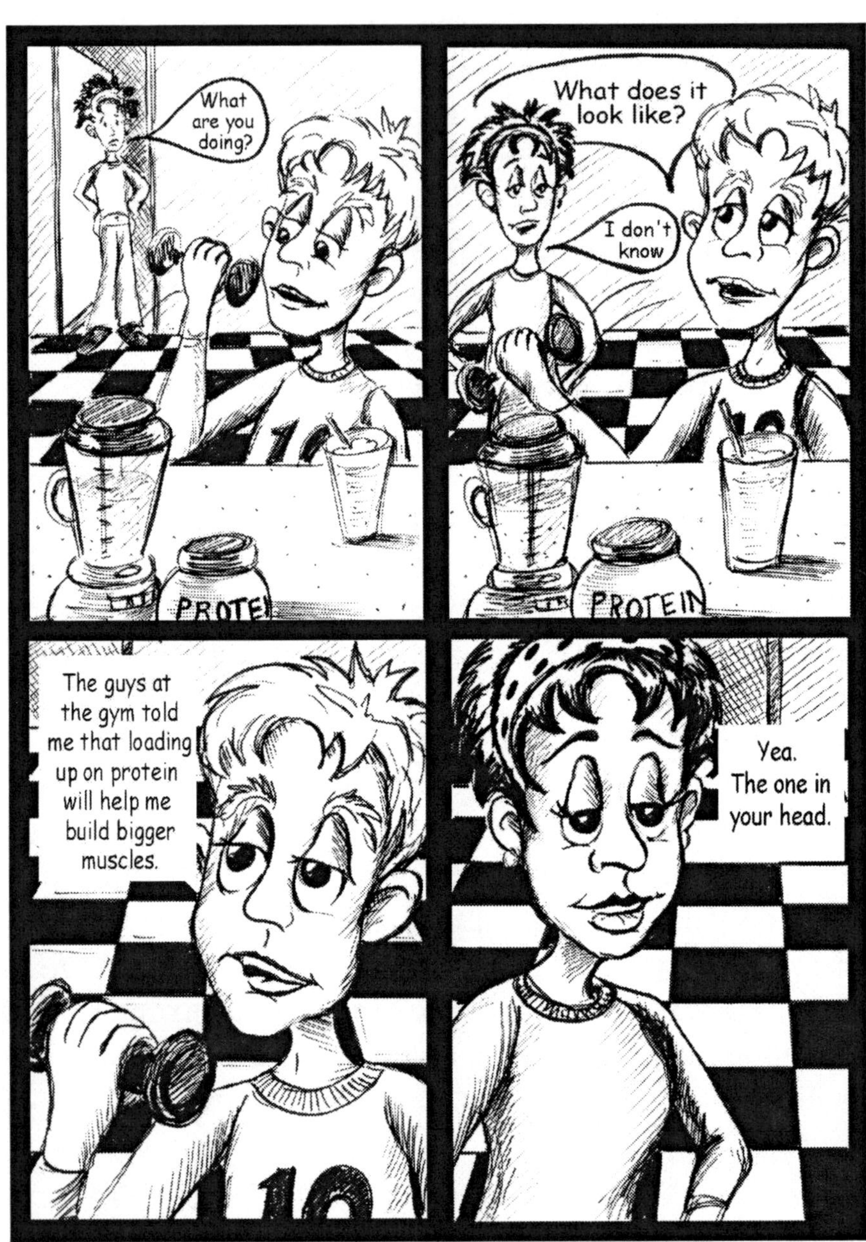

What are you doing?
What does it look like?
I don't know
The guys at the gym told me that loading up on protein will help me build bigger muscles.
Yea. The one in your head.

there are some experts that believe that the fiber in these types of manufactured products do not really contribute to better health. Getting fiber from fruits and vegetables are naturally better choices and should be consumed more often than processed types.

How much protein do we really need?

Chances are if you are eating a variety of foods every day you are not protein deficient, with the exception of people who are practicing vegetarianism incorrectly. Most of us get more than we really need and contrary to popular belief, that excess gets stored as fat just like other excess calories if they are not used up. The average person needs about 15% of their calories to come from protein. If you are vegetarian, it becomes critical that you study how to combine plant foods properly in order to get the high quality protein your body needs.

If you are an athlete or body builder, you may need a bit more, but not to the extent that you need to supplement your diet with extra through eating a very high protein diet or using high protein supplements. This is a very popular philosophy now but, sadly it has no real merit. In fact, taking in more protein than you need will not only turn to fat, it is very hard on your kidneys which need to process and filter all the protein metabolism by-products out of your system. Ever wondered why you need to drink tons of water when consuming high amounts of protein? Now you do.

The other danger of consuming too much protein is that it causes your body to become more acidic. There are many chemical reactions that occur in the body all the time to keep everything in balance, so knocking it out of balance can cause your system to take nutrients from your bones to try and neutralize the excess. This can lead to bone loss and *osteoporosis*, a condition in which your bones become fragile over time. You don't want your body in a more acidic state for many other reasons. It is believed that this state can contribute to all kinds of disease and problems.

It's a complicated process, but in any case, too much protein in your diet does not give you an athletic or weight loss edge. So, if you are thinking about going on a high protein, low or no carb diet, you might want to rethink your decision. If you can't stay on a program for a lifetime, it does not give you lasting results and in some cases can even hurt you.

What is a calorie?

Just as a car needs fuel to run, your body needs energy to keep you going. The fuel that food supplies is measured in units called calories. So, for example, 1 gram of carbohydrate or protein provides 4 calories while one gram of fat provides 9 calories.

The number of calories you need depends on your gender, your weight and your activity level. About 2/3 of the calories you consume go to keeping your bodily functions going. These activities include: keeping your body temperature stable, keeping your heart, lungs and brain functioning, and your digestive tract moving and digesting food. Your body is also constantly repairing tissue and regulating chemicals inside and outside your cells as well as making important hormones. The rest of the calories get used for physical activity. If more calories are consumed than can be used they are stored for later use in your liver and muscles. If you don't use them up, any excess will get stored as fat regardless of where the calories came from. This is our evolutionary insurance of survival.

It is a common mistake to skip meals in order to "save" calories or reduce weight. In actuality, you have to eat often to lose weight. If you get too hungry your brain tells your body to go into starvation mode and conserve whatever fuel you have left and lower your metabolism since it doesn't know when you will feed it again. What better reason NOT to get over-hungry. Obviously this means using common sense and eating small healthy meals rather than snacking on empty nutrient deficient calories.

What is your body telling you when you feel hungry? If you said it is telling you it needs food you wouldn't be completely correct. What it really is telling you is that your body needs nutrients. All calories are not created equal when it comes to sustaining life. So, if you eat a doughnut in response to your hunger pangs your body is going to tell you "oops, thanks for playing but that is not what I need". There is no nutritional value to a doughnut so now you are still looking for something to take care of that pesky hunger. Eat something nutritious and the feeling will undoubtedly go away. Listen to your body, it knows exactly what it needs!

What do vitamins do?

If you reach for a vitamin and mineral supplement when you are feeling tired or run down, there is probably a basic misunderstanding of what vitamins are, how they function and contribute to health. Vitamins are definitely important. They got their name because they are "vital to life" however, they do not provide any calories so they cannot directly provide energy. Vitamins contribute to health by regulating metabolism, supporting cells, and assisting all the bio-chemical processes that release energy from the foods we eat. Unlike foods, which are considered *macronutrients* vitamins are referred to as *micronutrients* because the body needs only very small amounts in comparison. In fact, the amount of actual vitamins you need could fit into an 1/8 of a teaspoon. That small amount is very powerful though and should get your respect.

Because of the way vitamins function in our bodies, it is generally best to get them from the various foods we eat rather than taking them in individual supplement form. For example, a fresh ripe apple has over 10,000 nutrients it in. They all work together to provide maximum nutrition to your cells. If you isolate one of those nutrients in a pill and take it, your body will not know how to digest it very well without the other 9,999 nutrients it originally came packaged with because it needs those other components to function optimally and be recognized as the nutrient that it is. That is why vitamin supplements come in such high doses. Your body can only use a very small percentage of the total amount in the pill because it is not well recognized in that isolated form. It's kind of like listening to a band without the drum section. It doesn't sound right and isn't complete right? Think of eating your vitamins through food as providing a healthy symphony to your cells complete with all the instruments that make it sound good, consequently providing harmony and balance for your health.

So, the fact is that the body recognizes vitamins from food much more efficiently and can utilize them in a healthy way. Whereas, it is difficult to regulate how much of any one nutrient you are absorbing from supplements. In fact, taking too much can be harmful to your health. In some cases, it is necessary to use "vitamin therapy" for short periods of time under medical supervision but it is not advisable to self prescribe.

If you eat a variety of foods that include lots of colorful fruits and veggies as well as lean protein sources and good carbs you should be fine in most cases. If you still feel you need to supplement your diet, try a whole food alternative like Juice Plus+® instead where the nutrition of a variety of nutrient dense fruits, vegetables and grains have been juiced, dried and concentrated into capsule form to give you that extra nutrition boost without the possible harmful long term side effects of high dose vitamins. And, because Juice Plus+® is simply whole food nutrition similar to juice without the water, salt, and sugar, your body knows what it is and can use all of its nutritional power.

How does fiber fit in?

Fiber is one of those awesome components of some foods that not only contributes to good health but can help regulate weight and keep cholesterol levels down. In fact, it is really the only natural way to eat low carb. It is definitely your friend and most of us probably need to increase the amount we eat. It is recommended that we get at least 25–35 grams per day. This is not hard to do if you eat lots of whole foods, meaning those that contain whole grains, skins, pulp and seeds. There are actually two types of fiber and both have their own benefits.

There is the type that you can see such as the examples I just mentioned. This is generally *insoluble* fiber. That means your body does not directly digest it so it doesn't contribute to calories in the diet. It is commonly referred to as "roughage" and speeds the passage of foods through the intestinal tract, promoting regularity. Metabolic waste is something you don't want lingering around too long because it can cause problems and increase risk of some cancers and disease. Plus, if you have a clear path to the intestinal wall you will absorb more of the nutrients you are eating since the intestinal wall is where most of the nutrients get absorbed into the bloodstream. If you are going to try and eat healthy it would be good to get the full benefit, don't you think?

The other type of fiber is called *soluble*. This type you generally can't see but is abundant in fruits, veggies, beans and some grains like oat, rice and corn bran. Soluble fiber, like the pectin in apples, turns to a gel in your body and helps mop up the bad cholesterol and transports it back to the liver for elimination. This helps you stay away from heart disease and other types of cardiovascular diseases. Soluble fiber may also help slow down the absorption of sugar into the bloodstream.

You need both kinds, so as long as you eat a variety of foods including lots of fruits, veggies and whole grains, you should be good to go. There are also some great whole grain breads, pastas, and cereals out there now that have much more fiber than their regular counterparts. Choose these products over the others whenever you can. It automatically has you eating low carb the healthy way. How about that?

Tips to increase your fiber

Choose cereals with 5 or more grams of fiber per serving.

Add 2–3 tbsp. of unprocessed oat, ground flaxseed or wheat bran to any cereal.

Choose soups with lentils, grains, beans, and vegetables.

Eat fresh fruit with skin on instead of having juice.

Prepare vegetables and potatoes with skin left on.

Choose dark green or bright colored vegetables and salad.

Add lentils, garbanzo, black, pinto, or kidney beans to a salad.

Choose brown rice over white.

Choose whole grain bread over white.

Don't be fooled by labeling, "enriched wheat flour" is basically white flour because the husks and bran which contain the fiber have been removed. It may look brown, but that is just coloring to make it look more like whole grain.

The importance of water

Our bodies are composed of about 2/3 water. Consequently our bodies depend on the constant replenishing of this vital fluid since it is involved in just about every bodily function there is. If you deprive your body of water, it has to take it from vital organs, muscles and other parts of your body in order to maintain normal functioning. It is smart to drink at least 1/2 your body weight (in ounces) of fresh clean filtered water every day whether you are thirsty or not and when you become an adult 64 ounces is minimum. Thirst is not a good indicator. In fact, by the time you feel thirsty you are probably pretty dehydrated.

What constitutes fresh clean water? While tap water is regulated and monitored closely, it can have things in it that your body really doesn't need causing YOU to be the filter of such things as tiny debris from pipes, small amounts of varying contaminants and lots of chlorine. It is hard to pinpoint everything that might be in your water source as it varies from location to location. Because your water is regulated, unwanted debris and things that could contaminate the water are checked all the time to make sure that they are kept at a minimum and will do no harm, however, it's better not to get them at all.

These "other things" can be the least of the problems associated with drinking tap water. Chlorine is really what I want to talk about here. It has already been established that chlorine causes cancer and probably contributes to all kinds of other health problems. Water districts are required to provide safe water, which means it has to be chlorinated in order to remain safe and sanitized.

Here is an analogy that fits. When you go to the store and buy a loaf of bread, it most likely comes wrapped in plastic or some other type of wrapper. Well, when you want to eat the bread you take a piece out of the wrapper rather than eating the wrapper with it right? Think of chlorine as a wrapper, you need it to come to you that

way for safety reasons, but you don't want it in your body.
So, what can you do? Buy a good water filter. A good
reputable company can tell you whether their filter gets
rid of chlorine and other contaminants. The filter should
also contain a good antimicrobial agent since water will
be sitting in it during times you are not using it, which
could breed bacteria. You will have to do some research,
but it is worth it! Wouldn't you rather buy and use a filter
than let your kidneys become one? Someone very smart
said that to me once and it made really good sense and
still does.

So what about bottled water? There are several problems
that can be associated with bottled water. Bottled water is
not as regulated as city water. This puts you in a position
of not really knowing what the standards are that the
company uses, how it is processed and where it comes
from. The plastic that the water comes in can also pose
health problems if you let the water get too warm, keep it
too long, freeze it, or drink from the same bottle
throughout the day. Because plastic is made from
petroleum (an oil product) it can have properties in it that
can leach into the water and be potentially harmful and
may even contribute to increased risk of some cancers.
And, if you continually drink from the same bottle, the
incidence of bacteria can multiply exponentially
throughout the day. In fact, studies have likened the
bacteria content of water bottles that have been used
consistently without cleaning them, to drinking toilet
water. Not a pretty picture, especially if you are trying to
do yourself a favor by drinking water throughout the day.

If you insist on drinking bottled water because of its convenience and taste, don't store it too long, leave it in warm places, freeze it, or drink from the same bottle all day.

Water that comes from a water cooler has some of these same problems but also comes with the added problem of cooler sanitation. It is not uncommon for water coolers to go without being cleaned and sanitized for long periods of time. Anytime you have a dark moist environment, there is potential for bacteria growth, YUCK! Besides, it is far less expensive to buy a good water filter than pay for expensive bottled water. The peace of mind and money you save will pay off in your pocket book as well as your health.

The average person loses about 10 cups of water every day. Here is how it adds up. You lose about 2 cups to perspiration, 2 cups to respiration (breathing) and about 6 cups to waste removal and if you exercise you can add quite a bit more. It is recommended that for every 15 minutes that you are exercising you should consume a few more ounces of additional water in order to perform well and prevent dehydration.

In case you aren't convinced, here are a few more good reasons to drink all that water. It suppresses appetite naturally and helps the body burn stored fat. It is the best form of natural *diuretic* (prevents fluid retention). It helps maintain muscle tone and regulates body temperature. It helps carry nutrients and oxygen to cells and removes wastes from your body. It cushions joints and protects organs and tissues, keeps your skin clearer and even helps ward off wrinkles by keeping your skin hydrated.

Believe it or not most people are walking around every day in a somewhat dehydrated state and don't even know it. Just 3% dehydration can slow down calorie burning and can even add up to an extra pound on the scale within about 6 months.

Water also contributes to better mental functioning and helps ward off headaches and constipation. Caffeine and alcohol will act as a diuretic and rob you of vital fluids. These beverages do not count toward water intake. High water content fruits and veggies can contribute up to 2 cups of your daily water intake but your best bet is to stay close to the water source and take a drink whenever you can, your body and good health will thank you for it. *Having said that, you can overdose on water also. This condition is called hyponutremia. It is more common in distance athletes. Drinking huge volumes of water can imbalance electrolytes in your system that help regulate minerals in the blood. This can be very dangerous, so be sensible. You can get too much of a good thing!*

Soda, the multipurpose liquid

According to the Center for Science in the Public Interest (CSPI), of the 85% of teens who drink soda between the ages of 13 and 18, boys consume an average of 32 ounces per day and girls consume about 23 ounces per day. The

CSPI is vigilantly advocating that the FDA put warning labels on soda pertaining to its contribution to obesity and tooth decay to mention just two possible consequences of drinking this sugary concoction.

Regular soda has been dubbed "liquid candy" because of the amount of sugar it contains. Diet is no better as it is simply a chemical cocktail. Can't live without it? Here are some good reasons why you might want to try.

I must preface this by saying that I don't know the source of these facts or whether they really even are facts, but if there is any truth to them, it is enough to steer me clear.

It has been speculated that you can:

1. Use cola to clean your toilet. Simply pour a can into the bowl and let the citric acid remove any stains.

2. Clean corrosion from car battery terminals. Pour a can of cola over the terminals and watch the fizz bubble away the corrosion.

3. Loosen a rusted on bolt by applying a cloth soaked in cola to the rusted area for several minutes.

4. Clean haze off your windshield with a cloth soaked in cola.

5. Use diet soda to clean the grease from your kitchen floor.

6. Cola can dissolve a nail in about four days.

7. Cola can disintegrate a raw steak in just two days.

Here is what I do know to be true. The active ingredient in cola is phosphoric acid and its Ph is 2.8 which is much more acidic than the Ph of your body. Making your body more acidic can cause lasting health effects and disease. Our bodies thrive better on foods that prevent acidity. It will also leach vital minerals from your bones as your body neutralizes the acid, which can start you on the path to osteoporosis. It doesn't matter if it is the diet version or the real thing. While the diet version doesn't contain 12 teaspoons of sugar, it does contain toxic artificial sweeteners. Still want your soda? Proceed at your own risk!

Are you fated to be fat?

The answer is no. Studies show that a susceptibility to be overweight can be higher in some due to many different factors. However, it is only a greater susceptibility not necessarily an inevitability. Statistics indicate that genetics, diet, lifestyle, and exercise habits all rate when it comes to probability so you can certainly tip the scale in your favor by adopting a healthy lifestyle that includes being active and eating right.

A word about smoking

Peer pressure can be a really strong influence on your choices during the teenage years. It might be cool right at first, but beware, some say quitting can be more difficult than kicking heroin addiction and it's not a joke or something to take lightly. Your decision to start may not be as easy when you decide to quit. Not only does it have an amazing way of separating you from your hard earned cash, it has serious negative health effects that could very well change your entire health profile and future. Never mind that it contains over a thousand carcinogens and that it deposits black tar in the most delicate part of your lungs which are responsible for oxygen transfer to your body and brain. You aren't going to look too cool dragging around an oxygen tank behind you wherever you go. And if you think I'm kidding go check out the respiratory or pulmonary ward in a hospital sometime, it's not pretty.

In any case, we are all products of the choices we make. It's easy to say no when you haven't started yet. Keep that monkey off your back, it's a lot easier than prying him off later. Believe me, you will have a brighter future for having made that decision. And, if you are reading this and already smoke, the best thing you can do for your health right now is to decide to quit. There are plenty of resources, products, and support groups to help. The good news is, your lungs have an amazing ability to regenerate and heal. Once off the cigarettes, in most cases, you can get your pink healthy lung tissue back in a relatively short time assuming you do it now, not in 20 or 30 years.

Main dishes

Beef fajitas

Makes 4

1 lb. grass fed skirt steak or top sirloin, cut into small strips

1 green pepper, seeded, cut into strips

1 red or orange pepper, seeded, cut into strips

1 large red onion, cut into strips

1 packet dry fajita seasoning

1/2 cup water

Cayenne pepper to taste

4 burrito size, whole wheat tortillas

Sour cream, optional

In a nonstick or lightly greased large skillet, sauté beef, peppers and onion until beef is cooked. Add packet of seasoning and water and cook down so that very little liquid remains. Add cayenne. Heat tortillas and divide fajita mixture evenly between the 4 tortillas, add sour cream if desired and enjoy. Serve with a green salad to make a nicely balanced meal.

The heat of a particular type of chili can vary greatly according to where it was grown and the conditions it was grown in. The hotter and drier the climate, the spicier the chili crop. Here are some hints for predicting chili's heat. Small chilies, like Serranos and jalapenos are generally spicier than larger ones like Anaheims or New Mexicans. Red varieties can be sweeter than green ones and dried chilies are often more flavorful but less hot than their fresh counterparts.

Another little known fact is that there is a potent chemical in chilies called capsaicin (pronounced capsaysin) that acts as a powerful pain reliever as well as an *anticoagulant*. An anticoagulant helps keep blood clots from forming, consequently allowing the blood to flow more freely through our systems. Just as you would rather drive a freeway that doesn't have traffic jams, you want your blood to flow freely so it can perform all the functions you need for good health such as transporting oxygen and nutrients to all your body tissues.

The powerful habanera from Mexico's Yucatan can be found dried in most supermarkets. Some may carry it fresh. If you can find it fresh that would be the preferred choice. The habanera is orange and lantern shaped. It is about the size of a walnut and is rated one of the hottest chili peppers there is. A little goes a long way so don't overdo it! If you can't find them or don't care for the hotter chilies, ask the produce manager to recommend an alternative.

Salmon with citrus habanera salsa

Serves 4

This easy dish can be made to look very impressive when served on a bed of greens that have been sprinkled with rice vinegar and served on some fluffy brown rice.

4 tomatoes, chopped

1/2 red onion, peeled and chopped

1 to 2 habaneras, seeded and chopped

1 tbsp. olive oil

1/2 tsp. salt

1/2 tsp. cumin

1/4 tsp. cinnamon

Juice of 3 oranges or 1/2 cup orange juice

4 (4–6 ounce) wild salmon fillets

2 tbsp. butter

Combine tomatoes, onion, and habanera in blender and purée until smooth. Heat oil in medium saucepan over medium heat. Pour in purée, salt, cumin and cinnamon and boil about 7 minutes. Pour in orange juice, reduce heat, stir and cook 1 minute longer. Melt 2 tbsp. butter in skillet over medium heat. Sear fish 2 minutes per side,

then reduce heat and cook 2 minutes more per side. Place
fish on plate or on top of greens and spoon sauce over
top of each fillet. Serve with brown rice and veggies.

Salmon is one of those wonderful foods that packs a good protein punch as well as a healthy dose of omega3 fatty acids. As mentioned in the demystifying fat section, omega3 fatty acids are very heart healthy. Eating 2 to 3 servings a week of foods high in omega3's can lower risk of cardiovascular disease.

Buying fish can be tricky though, and it is best to buy your fish wild, not farmed. Farmed fish is not the healthiest way to go as the fish have not been able to live a natural life. They start in a hatchery and end there with large numbers of fish in each pond. Having such a large population of fish together lends itself to disease, so the hatcheries may have to treat ponds with antibiotics and pesticides to keep illness down. All this gets into the meat and ultimately into you. Also, these fish do not get their natural food or exercise causing their meat to look whitish grey rather than the healthy pink they are in the wild. So, in order to make them look palatable they add pink color to restore a more natural look. Regulations now mandate that all fish be labeled if it is farmed and has color added. Your best bet is to avoid farmed varieties all together.

There can be some inherent problems with fish even from the wild due to mercury concentrations in the water. The best way to avoid high concentrations of mercury is to not buy all your fish from the same waters and avoid larger fish like swordfish and shark. These fish have had a longer time to accumulate mercury from the water and from the smaller fish they eat regularly. If you are a smart consumer, you can reap the healthful benefits from fish without the negatives. By all means don't avoid fish because of this information, use your knowledge to make smart decisions.

Flank steak jalapeno

Serves 4

3 jalapenos, seeded and sliced (for less heat
use 1–2)

4 garlic cloves, peeled

2 tsp. black pepper

1/4 tsp. salt

1/4 cup lime juice

1 tbsp. dried oregano

1/8 cup olive oil

1-1/2 lb. grass fed flank steak

Combine the jalapenos, garlic, black pepper, salt, lime
juice, oregano, and olive oil in a blender or food
processor and purée. Pour over steak in shallow roasting
pan and coat all the meat with sauce. Cover and marinate
in refrigerator 2 to 24 hours. Preheat grill or broiler. Grill
or broil 5 minutes per side for medium-rare, longer if you
like your meat cooked more. When done, let sit 5 minutes
before slicing. Cut in thin slices across grain of meat and
serve with a salad and veggies. Leftovers are great for
sandwiches and to add to salads!

*I mentioned previously that buying natural or organic
meat is really the only way to go. If you can find **grass***

fed beef, that will let you know that you are buying high quality natural beef. Specialty meat markets and whole food stores will carry it. Again, it will cost a bit more, but the cost is minimal when you consider the alternative.

Spicy mango chicken

Serves 4

4 boneless, skinless, free range chicken breasts

Salsa:

1 large papaya, peeled, seeded and diced

3 jalapenos, stemmed, seeded and minced (for less heat, use 1–2)

1/4 cup minced red onion

1/4 cup chopped cilantro

2 tbsp. lime juice

1 tbsp. olive oil

Bake chicken breasts in 350 degree oven for 30 to 40 minutes until done. Meanwhile combine all salsa ingredients in bowl. Toss thoroughly. Spoon generously over baked chicken and serve with brown rice and a green salad for a colorful nutritious meal.

Buying the right chicken will make all the difference to your health. Unfortunately, large production chicken farms have a disadvantage when it comes to healthful benefits because they are dealing with high volumes of chickens in small spaces. Again, anytime you have large populations, disease can be more prevalent which could mean antibiotic and pesticide treatment as well as other additives.

Read the label on your chicken, if it contains flavor enhancing broth put it back. These broths are preservatives that contain things like phosphates that are typically found in dishwashing liquid! If you stick with fresh, natural, free range, or organic chicken you know you are getting the best your money can buy. Plus you have the benefit of knowing that the chickens probably lived a much more humane life, which in my opinion is worth the extra money too.

Using herbs & spices

Herbs and spices are a wonderful way to enhance the flavor of your recipes. They are also a much healthier way to spice things up than tipping the salt shaker! The following guide will help you pair the right herb or spice with the right food but don't just stop there, be creative, not everything has been invented yet. Who knows, maybe YOU are the next great chef in the making!

Fresh herbs are becoming more widely available all the time. You can find them in just about every store and they can be fun and easy to grow right in your own home.

Whether you cut them from your own garden or buy fresh herbs from the produce department of your grocery store you will want to handle them with care to ensure maximum flavor and freshness. If you aren't going to use them right away, make sure you wrap them in damp paper towels, place them in a plastic bag and refrigerate until you are ready to use them. Of course it is best to use them right away if you can, but if not, taking this small precaution will help keep them fresh for a short time.

Cooking tip: When using fresh herbs in a cooked recipe, don't add them until close to the end of the cooking time to maintain their delicate flavor.

You can also use dried herbs and spices if you don't have access to fresh all the time. These can be a very convenient alternative as they keep much longer and can stand longer cooking times. Make sure you store your dried herbs and spices in an airtight container in a cool dry place. This will ensure that the flavors will stay fresher over time. You will also use quite a bit less when using dried as they are more concentrated that way. Check out appendix A in the back of the book for herbs and spices from A to Z.

What about additives & preservatives?

By now you know that eating artificial stuff isn't good for you. Additives are placed in foods for a lot of reasons. One of the main reasons is to lengthen the time it can be stored on the shelf without going bad. Sometimes they are added to make foods more appealing either by enhancing color, texture or taste. "Instant" foods have additives so that they can be made instantly.

There are over 3000 different government approved additives ranging from sugar and salt to even vitamins that are added to fortify food that normally wouldn't contain them. In fact, salt, sugar, corn syrup, pepper, baking soda, mustard, and vegetable colors account for about 98 percent of all additives that end up in our food supply. Although many additives are used in very small amounts, it is estimated that the average American consumes about 5 pounds of additives per year. If you include sugar in that number you have to increase that to 135 pounds per year! Yikes.

In most cases, additives add no nutritional value to food, and in some cases, can really be harmful to health. How do you know if you are eating lots of artificial ingredients and additives? If your diet consists mostly of processed and prepackaged foods you are getting a very unhealthy dose of the stuff every day.

The history of additive use includes quite a few that were originally thought to be safe. Some eventually caused health problems and were banned or only allowed to be used if a warning came on the label. Included on this list are artificial sweeteners, flavor enhancers, and artificial colorings. Some of these are believed to be responsible for some allergies and negative health effects. Again, your best bet is to steer clear of anything artificial whenever possible.

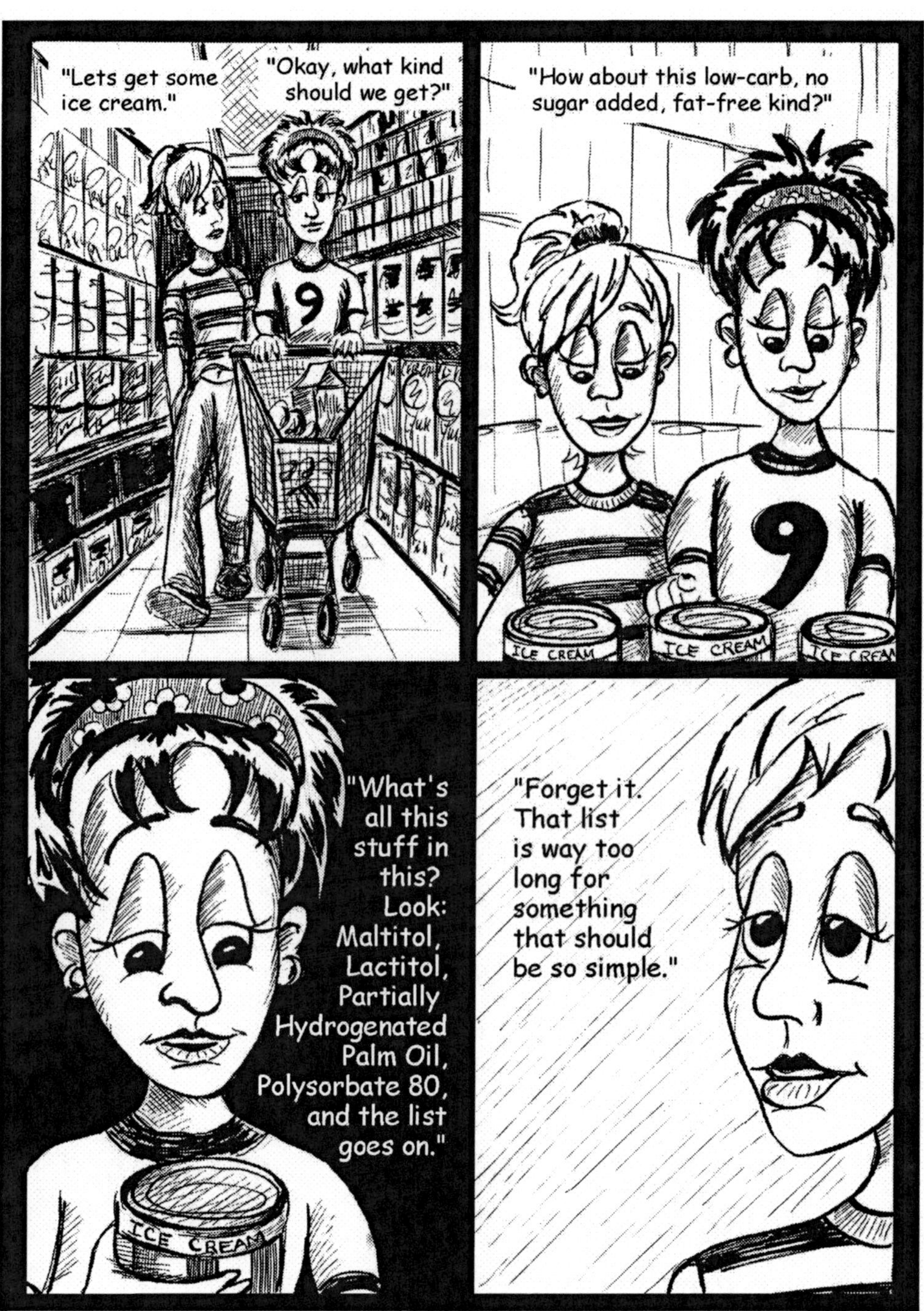

"Lets get some ice cream."
"Okay, what kind should we get?"
"How about this low-carb, no sugar added, fat-free kind?"
"What's all this stuff in this? Look: Maltitol, Lactitol, Partially Hydrogenated Palm Oil, Polysorbate 80, and the list goes on."
"Forget it. That list is way too long for something that should be so simple."
ICE CREAM
ICE CREAM
ICE CREAM
9

Desserts

Although some of these desserts may not seem healthy, natural ingredients and moderation are the keys to enjoying these treats occasionally. When we stick to what is natural, it is easier to live mindfully. We don't need everything to be microwave quick. We shouldn't have to rush life, squeezing it in between school and appointments then packaging it to go. Relax, slow down once in awhile and make some cookies…it's one of life's little pleasures.

Indulging in dessert once in awhile is not the problem, overindulging is.

Whole wheat oatmeal cookies

Makes 3-1/2 dozen

1 cup whole wheat flour

1 tsp. ground cinnamon

1 tsp. baking powder

1/2 tsp. baking soda

1/2 tsp. salt

3/4 cup light brown sugar

1/4 cup applesauce

2 egg whites

2 tbsp. butter, softened

2 tsp. vanilla

1-1/3 cup rolled oats

1/2 cup raisins, optional

1/2 cup chopped walnuts, optional

Preheat oven to 375 degrees. Lightly grease cookie sheets
or use nonstick baking sheets. Combine flour, cinnamon,
baking powder, baking soda and salt in medium bowl;
mix well.

Combine brown sugar, applesauce, egg whites, butter and
vanilla in large bowl; stir until mixed. Add flour
mixture; mix well. Stir in oats, raisins and nuts. Drop
rounded teaspoonfuls of dough, 2 inches apart, onto
prepared cookie sheets. Bake 10–12 minutes or until
golden brown. Cool on wire racks.

Light chocolate chip cookies

Makes 2 dozen

3-1/2 tbsp. brown sugar

3 tbsp. light corn syrup

1-1/2 tbsp. butter

1/2 tsp. vanilla

2 egg whites

2 tbsp. water

2/3 cup whole grain pastry flour

1/2 cup instant nonfat dry milk powder

1/2 tsp. baking soda

1/4 tsp. salt

1 cup rolled oats

1/2 cup chocolate chips

Combine first 4 ingredients in a medium bowl; beat at medium speed with electric mixer until light and fluffy. Add egg whites and water; beat well.

Combine flour, dry milk powder, baking soda and salt in medium bowl, stir well. Gradually add flour mixture to creamed mixture, mixing well. Stir in oats and chocolate chips.

Drop dough by level tablespoonfuls, 2 inches apart, onto lightly greased cookie sheets. Bake at 375 degrees for 9 to 11 minutes or until lightly browned. Cool slightly on cookie sheets before removing them onto wire racks.

Delectable chocolate brownies

Makes about 15

1/2 cup boiling water

1/2 cup unsweetened cocoa powder

1-1/4 cup whole grain pastry flour

1/2 cup sugar

1/2 cup brown sugar

1 tsp. baking powder

1/4 tsp. salt

4 egg whites, lightly beaten

1/3 cup applesauce

2 tsp. vanilla

1/2 cup chopped walnuts

Preheat oven to 350 degrees. Lightly grease 11X7 inch baking pan. Combine boiling water and cocoa in large bowl; mix until completely dissolved. Add flour, sugar, brown sugar, baking powder, salt, egg whites, apple sauce and vanilla; mix well. Fold in chopped nuts.

Pour batter into prepared pan. Bake 15–20 minutes or until brownies spring back when lightly touched. (*be careful not to overbake*) Cool in pan on wire rack; cut into bars.

Peanut butter cookies

Makes about 2 dozen

1-1/4 cup whole grain pastry flour

1/2 tsp. baking powder

1/2 tsp. baking soda

1/2 cup butter, softened

1/2 cup sugar

1/2 cup light brown sugar

3/4 cup natural peanut butter

1 egg

1 tsp. vanilla

Preheat oven to 350 degrees. Place flour, baking powder, and baking soda in small bowl.; stir to combine. Beat butter, sugar and brown sugar in large bowl with electric mixer at medium speed until light and fluffy. Beat in peanut butter, egg and vanilla. With a spoon or fork, gradually stir in flour mixture until well blended.

Roll heaping tablespoonfuls of dough into 1 inch balls. Place balls 2 inches apart on ungreased cookie sheets. Press criss-cross marks onto each ball with fork flattening to 1/2 inch thickness. Bake 15 minutes or until set. Let cookies cool and then remove with spatula and place on wire racks.

This rather unique summer dessert is as tasty as it is beautiful to look at. It is also very healthy. The berries are high in vitamin C and other antioxidants while the ricotta cheese is higher in calcium that any other cheese. You will surely impress your guests with this one!

Summer berry fantasy

Serves 8

1 bag (12oz.) frozen raspberries, thawed

1/4 cup plus 2 tbsp. sugar, divided

1 tbsp. lemon juice

2 cups sliced fresh strawberries

1 cup fresh raspberries

1 cup fresh blueberries

1 cup low-fat ricotta cheese

1 tsp. vanilla

1/2 tsp. almond extract

To prepare raspberry sauce, place thawed raspberries, 1/4 cup sugar and lemon juice in blender or food processor; process until smooth. Drizzle 3 tablespoons raspberry sauce onto each of 8 dessert plates.

Arrange 1/4 cup strawberries, 2 tablespoons raspberries and 2 tablespoons blueberries on top of sauce in creative pattern on each plate.

Place ricotta cheese, remaining 2 tbsp. sugar, vanilla and almond extract in blender or food processor and process until smooth. Spoon ricotta cheese mixture into pastry bag; pipe onto berries, using about 2 tbsp. of mixture on each serving. (Use star tip to make rosettes or various sizes of writing tips to drizzle mixture over berries instead) Be creative with this and have some fun!

Tip: If you don't own a pastry bag, spoon the cheese mixture artfully on top of fruit.

Peach sherbet

Makes 3 cups

1 (8 oz.) container plain low-fat yogurt

1/2 cup orange juice

1/4 cup honey

2 cups peaches, peeled and sliced or use frozen unsweetened peaches, partially thawed.

Place all ingredients in food processor or blender. Process until peaches are finely chopped. Pour mixture into 8 inch square pan; freeze until almost firm. Spoon back into food processor/blender and process until smooth but not thawed. Return mixture to pan and freeze until firm. Let stand at room temperature 10 minutes before scooping into serving dishes. Serve immediately.

Berry Frozen Yogurt

Makes about 7 cups

4 (16 oz.) packages unsweetened frozen blackberries, strawberries, or raspberries, thawed

1 (16 oz.) carton vanilla low-fat yogurt

3/4 cup milk

1/3 cup sugar

Place berries in food processor and blend until smooth. Combine berry purée with yogurt, milk and sugar in a bowl and stir well.

Either pour mixture into ice cream maker and proceed according to directions or, pour mixture into large bowl and freeze until almost firm. Scoop mixture back into food processor or blender and blend until smooth but not thawed. Return to bowl and freeze until desired consistency. Serve.

Pumpkin cheesecake

Serves 16

3/4 cup crushed graham crackers

1 (16 oz.) can pumpkin

2 cups low-fat ricotta cheese

2/3 cups sugar

3 tbsp. all purpose flour

1 tbsp. nonfat dry milk powder

1 tbsp. ground cinnamon

1 tsp. ground allspice

1 egg white

3/4 cup evaporated skimmed milk

1 tbsp. vegetable oil

1 tbsp. vanilla

Preheat oven to 400 degrees. Lightly grease 9-inch spring form pan. Pack bottom with graham cracker crumbs. Set aside. Combine pumpkin and ricotta cheese in food processor or blender; process until smooth. Add sugar, flour, milk powder, cinnamon, allspice, egg white, evaporated skimmed milk, oil, and vanilla; process until smooth.

Pour mixture into prepared spring form pan. Bake 15 minutes. Reduce oven temperature to 275; bake 1 hour and 15 minutes more. Turn off oven; leave cheesecake in oven without opening door one more hour. Remove from oven; cool completely on wire rack. Carefully loosen cheesecake from side of pan; remove side. Cover cheesecake with plastic wrap; refrigerate at least 4 hours before serving.

Fluffy chocolate mousse

Serves 8

This fluffy and nearly fat free mousse is lighter than most chocolate desserts and is so quick and easy to make!

1/3 cup, plus 2 tbsp sugar, divided

1/4 cup unsweetened cocoa powder

1 envelope unflavored gelatin

2 tbsp. coffee flavored liqueur, optional

2 cups milk

1/4 cup egg substitute

2 egg whites

1/8 tsp. cream of tartar

1/2 cup whipped cream

Combine 1/3 cup sugar, cocoa and gelatin in medium saucepan. Add liqueur; let stand 2 minutes to soften gelatin. Add milk; cook and stir over medium heat until sugar and gelatin are dissolved. Cool and stir in egg substitute; set aside. Beat egg whites in medium bowl with electric mixer until foamy. Add cream of tartar; beat until soft peaks form. Gradually add remaining 2 tbsp. sugar until stiff peaks form. Gently fold egg white mixture into cocoa mixture; fold in whipped cream.

Divide mixture evenly among 8 dessert dishes and
refrigerate until thickened.

Appendix A:
herbs & spices from A to Z

Allspice

This Jamaican berry can be used whole or ground. Add a few berries to chicken, beef or fish stock, pot roast or beef stew. Add ground allspice to mulled cider, fruit desserts and compotes and of course pumpkin pie.

Anise

This seed smells and tastes like black licorice. It works well in spice cakes, cookies and other desserts. Whole or ground anise seed also goes well in fruit dishes and applesauce. Add some to braised beef or cooked cabbage for an intriguing new taste.

Basil

This wonderful fragrant herb can easily be grown at home. It goes well in just about everything but is known for its use in adding flavor and aroma to Italian food. It blends especially well with tomatoes, olive oil and garlic. It also complements any type of meat, poultry, shellfish and vegetable. It is the main ingredient in pesto sauce. Basil is available at most grocery stores in the produce section and the leaves can be used as a flavorful addition to salad greens.

Bay leaf

Bay leaves are usually found whole and dried although you can find them powdered also. It is mostly used whole. If you use the dry whole leaves they need to be added at the start of the cooking process to give them time to release their flavor. You will want to remove them from the dish before serving, although some European traditions believe in leaving the bay leaf in and whoever gets it served with the meal is said to have good luck bestowed upon them.

Caraway

The flavor and aroma of this seed is most associated with rye bread although; it is used in many northern European and German main dishes and salads. Try caraway seeds in potato salad or coleslaw, cucumber salad, meatloaf or simply sprinkled over noodles. It does have a pungent strong flavor though that people either like or don't like.

Cardamom

This spice is used widely in Scandinavia and India. Its essence can be described as warmly sweet. It is very good with warm fruit dishes, baked apples and gingerbread yet it also seasons Swedish meatballs. It can be used in home made curry powder, and in sweet rice pilafs. Try using it in recipes that call for sweet potatoes, pumpkin and winter squash.

Cayenne

This spicy seasoning is made by grinding dried hot red chili peppers. It is an ingredient in chili powder and is used in Mexican, Indian, Chinese, and Cajun recipes. It is also good in marinades and barbecue sauces for meats, poultry and fish. Basically it can be added to anything you would like to give an extra kick to. It has even been known to be added to Mexican hot cocoa and chocolate. If you are not used to hot foods start with just a pinch.

Celery seed

This has a mild celery flavor due to the celery seeds it comes from. It can be used to enhance soup, fish chowders, tomato sauces, hot and cold potato dishes and stuffing.

Cilantro

Cilantro actually comes from coriander leaves. It is also called Chinese parsley. It resembles parsley but has flatter leaves and has a spicy aroma. Fresh cilantro is widely used in Mexican, Indian and Chinese cooking and can be found in just about every produce department. It doesn't retain its flavor very well when dried, so using it fresh is best. Add chopped cilantro to fresh salsa just before serving. It is also good chopped over grilled chicken or fish, sliced tomatoes, stir fry, legume, bean or rice salads or hot rice dishes.

Cinnamon

Who isn't familiar with cinnamon or doesn't enjoy the warm aroma of cinnamon wafting from the oven. It has traditionally been used in desserts and fruit dishes but less known is its inclusion in Moroccan and Greek chicken and beef dishes as well as rice pilafs. It is also a wonderful addition to winter squash, sweet potatoes, carrots and parsnips. Of course cinnamon sticks can be added to hot cider or fruit juices too.

Cloves

Everyone can identify the aroma of cloves. Whole dried cloves or ground cloves are typically combined with other sweet spices in apple desserts, gingerbread, and pumpkin pie. It can also enhance pea and bean soups, baked beans, chili, barbecue and tomato sauce, pork, ham and sweet potatoes.

Coriander seed

Whole or ground coriander seeds have a very distinct and pungent sweet fragrance. They differ wildly from coriander leaves, also known as cilantro and should not be mistaken for it. It is commonly used in Middle Eastern curry and Mediterranean dishes as well as being an ingredient in spice cakes and cookies. Use a pinch in soups, roast pork and salad dressings to spice them up a bit from the usual.

Cumin

Whole or ground cumin seeds go into making chili powder as well as curry powder so it is widely used from Mexico to the Middle East and India. Its flavor is best brought out when heated. Cumin complements beef and lamb, cooked carrots and cabbage, chickpeas, beans, lentils, and other legumes.

Dill seed

Dill seed is most known for its use in pickling. It is also good in salad dressings, sauces, and marinades. It couples well with fish and in cucumber, carrot, cabbage and potato salads as well as hot cooked cabbage, carrots, and potatoes.

Dill weed

Not to be confused with dill seed this feathery green leafed plant has a milder flavor than the seeds, but complements the same foods. Try adding a little to tuna or salmon salad, or to cottage cheese or yogurt for a savory dip or sauce.

Fennel seed

Like the vegetable it comes from, fennel seed has a mild licorice flavor. It is not as strong as anise. Fennel seeds go well with fish and shellfish, in Italian dishes and sauces, potato salad, and in rye bread.

Garlic

There are over 300 varieties of garlic grown around the world, but here in the United States we usually only see about 2 of them. One is called "early" and one "late". The early variety is harvested in mid-summer and the skins are whitish in color. The later harvest, which is harvested just a few weeks later, has a skin that is more pinkish in color. They taste much the same but the later harvest is denser and has a longer storage life. Garlic is best when used fresh and chopped or minced into recipes. Dehydrated, dry, powdered, and packed in oil are less than desirable alternatives as the taste doesn't translate as well. In Middle Eastern and Mediterranean countries, India and China, garlic is practically indispensable to their cooking while in Scandinavia and Britain, it is almost completely ignored. Almost anything is enhanced with the taste of fresh garlic, assuming you like the taste. It is great in pasta, to flavor meats and shellfish, added to salad dressing and sauces and used to flavor vinegar and oil. To make low-fat garlic bread, bake some cloves in the oven for 15 to 20 minutes until soft then squeeze the softened garlic flesh onto bread and spread like butter.

Ginger

In its fresh form ginger looks like a finger root. It is neither an herb or a spice but it is used as a seasoning. It has a light tan skin with yellowish flesh. You have to peel it before using it and it is generally grated or sliced. Fresh ginger will keep in the freezer for months if wrapped well and there is no need to thaw before using. Ginger has a sweet pungent flavor and is commonly used in Japanese dishes, marinades for chicken or fish, stir-fries, and fruit salad dressings.

Ground ginger

In its dried, ground form, ginger is most commonly used in baked goods such as gingerbread, spice cake, and pumpkin pie. However, it can also enhance braised poultry or meat, soups and stews, stuffing, cooked carrots, winter squash, sweet potatoes, and baked or stewed fruit. Try sprinkling it on grapefruit or rice pudding for a variation on taste.

Mace

Mace has a similar flavor to nutmeg but is a bit stronger because it comes from the dried, ground outer coating of the nutmeg berry. It can be used in the same way as nutmeg and is the classic spice for pound cake.

Marjoram

Also called sweet marjoram, this herb is closely related to oregano but has a more delicate flavor. It is especially good in tomato sauce and other tomato-based dishes. It is great with cooked lentils and beans, summer squash, potatoes, fish, lamb and veal.

Mint

Fresh mint leaves add zest to sweet dishes such as fruit salads and fruit soups, melon, berries, and cold fruit beverages. It is often used as a fragrant garnish. It can also be used with cooked carrots or peas, in fresh pea soup or chilled yogurt soup, with lamb and in cold grain salads, such as Tabbouleh. Its refreshing characteristics make this a particularly popular herb in warmer months.

Mustard

Mustard can be used whole in its seed form, ground dry, or in its prepared form which is most commonly used as a condiment for sandwiches, hot dogs and salads. It contributes a savory, spicy flavor. It is often used to enhance sauces for meat and fish, marinades and salad dressings, chutneys, pickles and relishes. It also complements fish and seafood salads, cooked spinach and cabbage family vegetables such as Brussels sprouts and cauliflower.

Appendix A

Nutmeg

This sweet spice is a favorite in fruit desserts and baked goods. Nutmeg can be freshly ground from the dried berry with a small grater however, most people buy it already ground. A pinch of nutmeg also enhances braised or stewed meats and poultry, white sauce, cooked spinach, broccoli, cauliflower, and carrots.

Oregano

This quintessential aromatic Italian herb is wonderful in tomato-based dishes of all kinds. What is less known is its use in Greek and Mexican cooking. Add it to sauces, salad dressings, soups or marinades. It also seasons baked fish, grilled poultry, mushrooms, green beans, and summer squash very nicely.

Paprika

Like cayenne, paprika is made by drying and grinding peppers, but is made from less pungent peppers and has a warmly sweet, rather than a hot, flavor. It is widely used in Spanish and Hungarian dishes. Rub poultry with paprika before roasting to add color and flavor. Sprinkle fish with it before broiling or baking. Add it to chowders, salad dressings and whenever a touch of color is needed. It goes well on top of pale dishes and vegetables such as potatoes, cauliflower or puréed soups to add color.

Parsley

This is the most widely available of all the fresh herbs and is used in a variety of different applications. It comes in both a flat-leaf and curly-leaf form which makes it very versatile and pleasing as a garnish and in cooking. Most people don't eat parsley when it comes as a garnish yet it has a very refreshing bite that will actually freshen breath after a meal better than a mint. When cooked it adds a boost of vitamin C to the dish as well as a spicy flavor. Toss in some freshly chopped parsley just before serving soups and stews, vegetables, pasta, grains, and eggs. Try sprinkling it over poached, baked or grilled meat, chicken, or fish. Adding it to salads and dressings adds color and flavor as well. Since fresh parsley is so widely available, stay away from the dried version as it is virtually flavorless.

Pepper

Did you know that pepper doesn't just come in black and white? There are a variety of different kinds of pepper corns including red and pinkish colored ones. The most commonly used are the black and white varieties. Black pepper comes from immature berries with their natural coating intact whereas white pepper berries are fully ripe and have had the outer layer removed. Why white pepper? To enhance pale foods without adding black specks to it such as mashed potatoes. It is best to buy whole pepper corns and grind them as needed as once they are ground they can lose their flavor pretty quickly.

Appendix A

Rosemary

This fragrant herb looks a bit like an evergreen sprig. It can be used to season chicken, lamb, pork, salmon and tuna, tomato sauces and soups, potatoes, mushrooms and peas. Adding it to bread before baking contributes an aromatic twist as well. When you are using fresh rosemary, it is necessary to chop and crush it thoroughly, as its needle-like leaves are quite hard. Even dried rosemary needs to be crushed or crumbled in order for it to release its true flavor.

Saffron

The most expensive of spices, saffron comes from a particular species of crocus. The spice is sold as "threads"—the whole stigma of the flower, or dried and in powdered form. Just a pinch is needed to add brilliant yellow color and an exotic, slightly bitter flavor to foods. It pairs well with seafood, poultry, Spanish, Italian, or Indian dishes, sauces and soups. It is commonly used in dishes such as paella, risotto and rice pilaf. Saffron should be dissolved in a small amount of warm water, a teaspoon or less will do, before adding it to a dish.

Sage

This seasoning is most known for its use in poultry stuffing. Sage is sold as whole leaves or crumbled and has a bold flavor and aroma. Try it with any type of poultry, pork, veal, or ham. It is also good in cheese sauces, legume or vegetable soups and seafood chowder, with cooked mushrooms, lima beans, peas, tomatoes, or eggplant.

Summer savory

This slightly peppery herb goes particularly well with vegetables, and is especially good with fresh or cooked green beans. It pairs well with peas, cabbage, Brussels sprouts, potatoes, legumes and in salad dressings. You can also use it to enhance poultry, fish, lamb, pork and cooked fruit.

Tarragon

This seasoning is essential to French cooking. It has a faint undertone of anise or licorice and can easily overpower other herbs so must be used carefully. Tarragon makes a great seasoning for poached, baked, or broiled fish or poultry, shellfish such as crab or shrimp and eggs. Try using a little in vinaigrette and other salad dressings, cooked potatoes, peas, asparagus, carrots, mushrooms and tomatoes.

Thyme

This herb is very versatile and though quite strong in flavor, it is compatible with many foods and is essential in Creole recipes. Add a little thyme to tomato sauce,

Appendix A

vegetable soup, clam and other seafood chowders, beef stew or pot roast, poultry stuffing, and cooked vegetables such as summer squash and green beans.
(The Wellness Encyclopedia of Food and Nutrition: How to Buy, Store and Prepare Every Variety of Fresh Food, 1992)

Appendix B:

measurement conversions

You will need some tools to use as a guide when it comes to measuring and converting between metric and traditional weights and measures.

Traditional (imperial) measures

3 teaspoons (tsp.) = 1 tablespoon (tbsp)

1/4 cup = 2 ounces

1/2 cup = 4 ounces

3/4 cup = 6 ounces

1 cup = 8 ounces

2 cups = 16 ounces =1 pint

2 pints = 32 ounces =1 quart

2 quarts = 64 ounces = 1/2 gallon

4 quarts = 128 ounces =1 gallon

Volume & weight

Americans traditionally use cup measures for liquid and solid ingredients. The chart below provides a guide for

Appendix B

converting measurements from the U.S. customary system, which is used throughout this book, to the metric system.

ml stands for milliliter

mg stands for milligram

g stands for gram

F stands for Fahrenheit

C stands for Celsius

Volume equivalents

Usually when we talk about volume measurements we are talking about liquid measurements.

1/4 tsp. = 1 ml

1/2 tsp. = 2 ml

1 tsp. = 5 ml

2 tsp. = 10 ml

1 tbsp. = 15 ml

1/4 cup = 60 ml

1/3 cup = 80 ml

1/2 cup = 120 ml

3/4 cup = 180 ml

1 cup = 240 ml

2 cups = 1 pint = 480 ml

4 cups = 1 qt = 950 ml

Dry weight equivalents

Usually when we talk about dry weight equivalents we are talking about measuring things like flour, sugar, salt etc. and it can depend on how dense what you are measuring is. For example take the ingredients below.

Notice that even though we use 1 cup as the standard, if we use grams things change a bit. Don't worry, if a recipe calls for grams they will tell you how many to use for each ingredient.

This information actually gives you a head start on your high school chemistry, how about that!

1 cup bread crumbs=140 grams

1 cup baking cocoa=80 grams

1 cup flour=140 grams

1 cup granulated (table) sugar=200 grams

1 cup powdered sugar=120

1 cup wheat germ=120 grams

Notice how the ingredients that seem more concentrated like cocoa and powdered sugar equal less grams?

Weight conversions

You will most likely run across these measurements when you are using things like meat or fish in your recipes. It will sure be helpful in chemistry class too! (Please note that due to fractional equivalents, ounces and grams do not convert precisely).

1 oz = 28g

2 oz = 57g

4 oz (1/4 lb) = 114g

5 oz = 142g

6 oz = 170g

8 oz (1/2 lb) = 227g

12 oz (3/4 lb) = 340g

14 oz = 397g

15 oz = 425g

16 oz (1 lb) = 450g

Temperature

Fahrenheit	Celsius
325	165
350	175
375	190
400	205
425	220
450	230

Again, here is a situation that probably won't occur unless you are cooking in another country other than the U.S. or using a foreign cookbook.

If you find yourself in higher altitude than 6000 feet, you also need to adjust your cooking temperature and time. Pay attention when a recipe mentions this as failure to adjust will result in a less than stellar product and that could be embarrassing to say the least! Usually this applies to things you are baking.

Appendix C:

Ingredient substitution list

Sometimes you want to make a recipe but you don't quite have all the ingredients the recipe calls for. Here is a list of substitutions you can use instead.

1 tsp. Baking powder:

1/4 tsp. baking soda plus 5/8 tsp. cream of tartar

Or   1/4 tsp. baking soda plus 1/2 cup buttermilk

1 cup Bread crumbs

3/4 cup cracker crumbs

1 cup Brown sugar

1 cup white sugar plus 2 tbsp. molasses

1 cup Butter

1 cup margarine

Or   7/8 cup vegetable oil

Or   7/8 cup butter flavored shortening

1 cup Buttermilk

1 cup plain yogurt

Or   1 tbsp. lemon juice stirred into milk to make 1 cup; let stand 5 minutes

(never use milk that has been in the frig too long and is sour; its spoiled)

6 squares or 6 ounces Chocolate, semisweet, melted

1 cup semisweet chocolate chips, melted

Or   1 ounce unsweetened chocolate plus 4 tsp. sugar

1 ounce Chocolate, unsweetened

1 square or 3 tbsp. unsweetened cocoa powder plus 1 tbsp. butter

Or   3 tbsp. unsweetened cocoa plus 1 tbsp. butter

1 cup Coconut cream

1 cup whipping cream

1 cup sweetened Condensed milk

Dissolve 1 cup plus 2 tbsp. dry milk powder plus 1/2 cup warm water plus 3/4 cup sugar

1 tbsp. Cornstarch

2 tbsp. flour

Or   2 tsp. quick tapioca

Or   2 egg yolks

1 cup Corn syrup

1-1/4 cup light brown sugar plus 1/3 cup water

Or   7/8 cup honey (baked goods will brown more)

Appendix C

1 cup Corn syrup, dark

> 3/4 cup light corn syrup mixed with 1/4 cup light molasses

1 cup Cream, light

> 3 tbsp. melted butter plus 3/4 cup milk

Or   1 cup evaporated milk

1/2 tsp. Cream of tartar

> 1-1/2 tsp. lemon juice or vinegar

1 Egg

> 1/4 cup egg substitute

1 cup Flour, all-purpose

> 1 cup whole wheat flour

Or   1 cup whole grain pastry flour

1 cup Flour, self rising

> 1 cup sifted all-purpose flour plus 1-1/2 tsp. baking powder and 1/2 tsp salt

1 clove garlic

> 1/8 tsp. garlic powder

1 tbsp. Herbs, fresh

> 1/2 to 1 tsp. dry herbs

1 cup Lard

> 2 cups shortening

1 tsp. Lemon juice

> 1/2 tsp. vinegar

1 tbsp. Maple sugar

> 1 tbsp. granulated sugar plus a dash of maple extract

3/4 cup Maple syrup

> 3/4cup maple flavored syrup

Or   3/4 cup corn syrup

Or   1 cup sugar and increase liquid in recipe by 3 tbsp

1 large Marshmallow

> 10 minis

1 cup Milk, whole

> 2 tsp melted butter plus 1 cup fat-free milk or water

Or   equal parts evaporated milk and water

Or   1 cup nonfat dry milk plus 2 tsp. melted butter

1 cup Molasses (in baking) omit baking soda; use baking powder

> 1 cup sugar

Appendix C

1 tbsp. prepared mustard

> 1/2 tsp. mustard seed

1 tsp. pumpkin spice

> 1/4 tsp. nutmeg, 1/4 tsp. ginger, 1/2 tsp. cinnamon

1 cup Ricotta cheese

> 1 cup cottage cheese

1 cup Sugar, granulated

> 13/4 cups powdered sugar for uses other than baking

1 cup Sugar (in baking)

> 7/8 cup honey plus a pinch of baking soda

1 cup Sugar (in baking bread)

> 1 cup honey plus a pinch of baking soda

1 cup Sugar (in main dishes)

> 3/4 cup honey

1 cup Sour cream

> 1 cup plain yogurt
>
> 3 tbsp. melted butter stirred into 7/8 cup butter-milk

1 pound Tomatoes

> 3 medium tomatoes

Or   3/4 cup tomato sauce (6 ounces)

Or   1/4 cup tomato paste (2 ounces)

3 cups Tomato juice

> 2-1/2 cups water plus 6 ounces tomato paste plus 3/4 tsp. salt and dash of sugar

8 ounces Tomato sauce

> 2/3 cup water plus 1/3 cup tomato paste

1 cup Vegetable oil

> 1 cup applesauce

1 cup Whipping cream as liquid

> 1/3 cup melted butter plus 3/4 cup milk

1 cup Whipping cream, whipped

> 2 cups thawed whipped topping

Or   Chill 13 ounces evaporated milk (until ice crystals form); add 1 tsp. lemon juice, whip

1/2 cup Wine, dry

> 2 tbsp sherry or port

Index

Measurement conversions 179
Mint 173
Mousse, fluffy chocolate 164
Muffin, apple cinnamon 47
Mustard 173

N
Nachos 75
Nutmeg 174

O
Omelet, open faced Spanish 23
Open faced Spanish omelet 23
Organic & Natural, why choose it? 55
Oregano 174
Oxygen is a bad thing? 89

P
Pancakes, blueberry with spicy blueberry syrup 20
Pancakes, perfect 19
Paprika 174
Parsley 175
Pasta salad, spring vegetable 81
Peach sherbet 160
Peanut butter cookies 157
Pepper 175
Perfect pancakes 19
Ph scale 38
Pita pizza 51
Pizza, pita 51
Potato crisps 73
Potatoes, creamy garlic mashed 113
Protein, how much do we really need? 123
Pumpkin cheesecake 162
Pumpkin spice smoothie 15

T

About the Author

Corie Goodson, MPH, CHES has
been interested in human
biology and health for as long as
she can remember. Even before
she started on her health degree
she was reading everything she
could get her hands on
regarding health issues. She
comes from a long genetic
history of cancer and stroke on

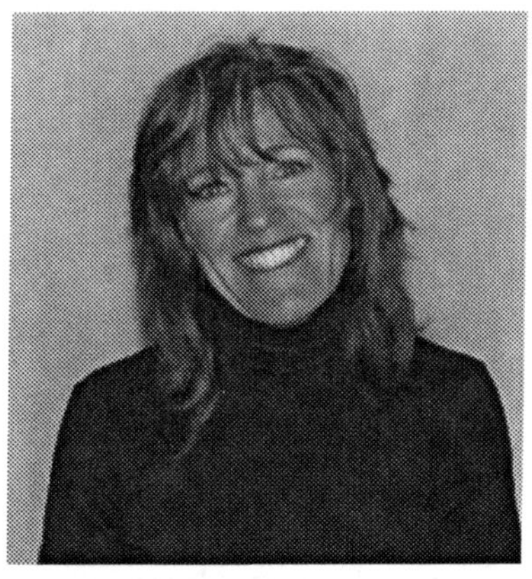

both sides of her family and so has been determined to
improve her odds by learning how prevention can tip the
scale in the right direction.

After earning a Bachelor's of Science degree in
Community Health Education she worked as a health
educator within several Health Maintenance
Organizations. Her primary job was to teach clients how
they could turn their health around through diet and
lifestyle after they had already become sick.
Unfortunately, trying to fix what was already broken was
extremely frustrating. She went on to get her Master's
degree in Public health and taught health and biology at
the community college level for several years.

In 2001 she decided to become a wellness speaker and
community health educator. Pursuing prevention and
educating are her true passions. With teen health being
such an important issue and the reality that the outlook is

not promising for future generations unless there is massive change, the idea for this book was born. "Kids today have too many of their own choices, many of them, unhealthy ones". Physical education is being taken out of schools while specialty coffee houses and vending machines are creeping in. Fast food is commonplace in school cafeterias now leaving the kids in charge of their choices, not the school dietitians.

Computers are standard equipment in every teen's life today making them more sedentary. It is estimated that the average teen spends more than 20 hours a week between the computer screen and the TV. Nutrition education is virtually nonexistent in most schools. With over 40,000 negative health messages being bombarded on teens annually, it looks like a long road uphill to change. Corie decided it was a road worth taking, even if it meant educating people one at a time.

This book is intended to be a fun vehicle that can educate and be entertaining as well as reintroduce the joy of cooking to this future generation of leaders. Corie believes that teaching prevention is the key to a healthier future. Small steps can add up to big results and a little education can go a long way toward that end.

About the Artist

Julie Malfitano grew up at the base of the Rocky Mountains in Longmont Colorado. From the instant she could hold a pencil Julie has dedicated every spare moment drawing anything and everything that came to mind. Her favorite subjects have always been whimsical cartoon characters and fairytale creatures, but she also adores painting classical portraits of children and families in natural settings.

Julie had always planned to pursue a career as a commercial artist and in 1996 she graduated from the Art center of Albuquerque with a degree in Advertising Art. Because of her diversity and ability to render art in numerous mediums and styles, she became very successful but eventually became stifled by the nature of the business and longed for more creative freedom and flexibility.

In the year 2001 with the loving support of her husband, she left advertising behind and began working as a freelance portrait artist and illustrator where she could freely express herself and spend more time with her family. Despite the cut in income and a few lifestyle adjustments, it is a decision Julie has never regretted. Every day brings new adventures carried on the wings of her two beautiful children who constantly inspire her and her loving husband who never stops believing in her.

References

About Southern U.S. Cuisine, "Ingredient Substitution List" 2004

Archives of Pediatric & Adolescent Medicine 1996; 150: 81–86

Archives of Pediatric & Adolescent Medicine 2000; 54: 203–287

Balch, P. A., CNC., & Balch, J. F., M.D. (2000). _Prescription for Nutritional Healing_ (3rd ed.). New York: Avery

Berenson, G., (2004, June). Epidemiology of Essential Hypertension in Children. _Pediatric Hypertension,_ pp. 121–142

Bogalusa Heart Study; National Heart Lung and Blood Institute (NHLBI) 2002

Center for Science in the Public Interest (CSPI)

Gale Encyclopedia of Children & Adolescents, Gale Research 1998

Gottfried, S., Ph.D. (1994). _Human Biology_. Montana: Mosby

Here's Health, April (1996). p72, Tower Publishing Services, Tower House.

International Journal of Obesity 1999; 23 (supp 2) S2-S11

Journal of the American Dietetic Association, 1999

Margen, S., & "Eds." of The University of California at Berkley WELLNESS LETTER. (1992). _The Wellness Encyclopedia of Food and Nutrition: How to Buy, Store, & Prepare Every Variety of Fresh Food_. New York: Random House

Pediatrics 1998; 101 (3) 497–504

That's My Home "Ingredient Substitution List" 2004

Webb, D., Ph.D., R.D. & Male Smith, S., M.A., R.D. (1995). Foods for Better Health: *Prevention & Healing of Diseases.* Illinois: Publications Intl. Ltd.

Printed in the United States
51124LVS00002B/1-102